0194630

KT-527-992

A Le...

WITHDRAWN

WITHDRAWN

WITHDRAWN

WITHDRAWN

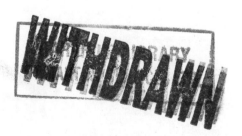

WITHDRAWN

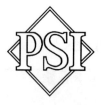

Policy Studies Institute (PSI) is one of Europe's leading independent research organisations undertaking studies of economic, industrial and social policy and the workings of political institutions.

PSI is a registered charity, run on a non-profit basis, and is not associated with any political party, pressure group or commercial interest.

PSI attaches great importance to covering a wide range of subject areas with its multidisciplinary approach. The Institute's researchers are organised in groups which currently cover the following programmes:

Crime, Justice and Youth Studies – *Employment* – *Ethnic Equality and Diversity* – *Family Finances* – *Information and Citizenship* – *Information and Cultural Studies* – *Social Care and Health Studies* – *Work, Benefits and Social Participation*

This publication arises from the Social Care and Health Studies Group and is one of over 30 publications made available by the Institute each year.

Information about the work of PSI and a catalogue of publications can be obtained from:

Publications Department, Policy Studies Institute, 100 Park Village East, London NW1 3SR

A LEADING ROLE FOR MIDWIVES?

Evaluation of Midwifery Group Practice Development Projects

Isobel Allen
Shirley Bourke Dowling
Sandra Williams

POLICY STUDIES INSTITUTE

PUBLISHING

The publishing imprint of the independent
POLICY STUDIES INSTITUTE
100 Park Village East, London NW1 3SR
Tel. 0171 468 0468   Fax. 0171 388 0914

© **Policy Studies Institute**

ISBN 0 85374 706 7
PSI Report 832

Reprinted 1997

PSI publications are available from:
BEBC Distribution Ltd, P O Box 1496, Poole, Dorset BH12 3YD

Books will normally be dispatched within 24 hours. Cheques should
be made payable to BEBC Distribution Ltd.

Credit cards and telephone/fax orders may be placed on the
following freephone numbers:
FREEPHONE   0800 262260
FREEFAX   0800 262266

Booktrade representation (UK and Eire):
Broadcast Books, 24 De Montfort Road, London SW16 1LZ
Tel. 0181 677 5129

PSI subscriptions are available from PSI's subscription agent:
Carfax Publishing Company Ltd,
P O Box 25, Abingdon, Oxford OX14 3UE

Laserset by Policy Studies Institute
Printed in Great Britain by Redwood Books, Trowbridge, Wiltshire

Contents

Tables

Acknowledgements

This study was commissioned and funded by South East Thames Regional Health Authority (now NHS Executive: South Thames) as an evaluation of three Midwifery Group Practice Development Projects set up by the Regional Health Authority.

The report presents an independent evaluation by Policy Studies Institute of the three midwifery group practices. We were greatly helped and supported throughout by a steering group established by the Regional Health Authority which had a broad membership representing different professional and academic interests. We would like to thank all members of the steering group: Ainna Fawcett-Henesy, Dr Gillian Dalley, Dr Leslie Davidson, Karlene Davis, Diane Garland, Dr David Garrioch, Kate Harmond, Paul Lewis, Dr Marc Rowland, Professor Terry Stacey and Dr Michael Vaile, most of whom were members throughout the evaluation. We would like to give particular thanks to Frances Pickersgill who coordinated the steering group and gave invaluable support and advice to the researchers.

We would like to thank the members of the three midwifery group practices for all their cooperation and help during the monitoring and evaluation period. The report draws attention to the workload of the pilot project teams, who were not only expected to deliver high quality innovative services as a model of practice for others to follow, but were operating under tight time constraints and the close scrutiny of external independent evaluators who needed them to supply accurate data on their activities.

We are also grateful to the GPs and consultant obstetricians in the three areas who spared the time to be interviewed by us and to give us their views.

Our major thanks go to the women who had babies with the midwifery group practices, most of whom were interviewed before and after the birth of their babies. Their views and experience reported in this evaluation add an important dimension to the continuing debate about the delivery of maternity services.

The study was designed and directed by Isobel Allen. Shirley Bourke Dowling was responsible for organising most of the field-work with the women and the professionals, and for the collection, processing and analysis of the data from the midwifery group practices. Sandra Williams was closely involved at a number of key stages of the evaluation, particularly in analysing the views and experience of the midwives and most of the work on resources. The three authors of the report were all involved in interviewing and the analysis and writing up of the data. Isobel Allen wrote the Discussion of Findings.

Kate Tomlinson was involved in the initial stages of the evaluation, particularly in the design of research instruments. Mary Ruth Haydon and Marion Kumar conducted many of the interviews with women and GPs and Mary Ruth Haydon was responsible for much coding and analysis of data. Anna Thomas conducted some interviews and Anna Grey helped with coding questionnaires.

Penny Swann played a major role in the collection and control of the monitoring data supplied by the midwifery group practices. Karen MacKinnon was responsible for the computing and preparation of tables and her help was much appreciated in the computer analysis of the data.

Chapter 1

Introduction

This report looks at the provision of maternity services at a time when providers and purchasers alike are responding to the recommendations of the report of the Expert Maternity Group, *Changing Childbirth* (Department of Health, 1993). Policy Studies Institute (PSI) was commissioned by the then South East Thames Regional Health Authority (SETRHA) to evaluate three midwifery group practices (MGPs) and to assess the effectiveness of these pilot projects in offering a model for the organisation, or reorganisation, of service delivery which could be replicated elsewhere.

Background

In March 1992, the House of Commons Health Select Committee reported on maternity services and concluded that 'a medical model of care' should no longer drive the service and that women should be given an opportunity to exercise choice in the type of maternity care they received. In response to the Select Committee's report the Government established an expert committee: 'To review policy on NHS maternity care, particularly during childbirth, and to make recommendations'. The Expert Maternity Group was set up in 1992 under the chairmanship of Lady Cumberlege and reported in 1993.

The Secretary of State for Health welcomed the Expert Maternity Group's Report, *Changing Childbirth*, which endorsed and amplified the views expressed in the Health Select Committee's report: that maternity services should be designed to allow women more control over their care, choice of treatment and place of delivery, and greater continuity of care. Laying out the next steps the Government encouraged the initiation of discussion locally and nationally on the changes needed in maternity services.

The midwifery group practice pilot projects

South East Thames Regional Health Authority (SETRHA) had already responded to the publication of the Health Select Committee's Report on

1

Maternity Services by initiating local discussions. In 1992 SETRHA had sponsored a Consensus Conference on maternity services for the future (SETRHA, 1992). Endorsing the views of the Health Select Committee, a major recommendation of this conference was that autonomous midwifery group practices should be established, with responsibility for the care of women from initial assessment to delivery and beyond. It was envisaged that the pilot projects would aim to provide high quality and safe maternity services in a community-centred location which would enable women to have choice, continuity of care and carer, and direct access to a midwife.

The South East Thames Nursing and Quality Directorate invited bids from providers of maternity services who wished to establish woman-centred care and delivery schemes in midwifery group practices. SETRHA stipulated that the pilot sites must fulfil the following criteria:

- *Organisation:* they were required to have 24-hour cover available; client-held records; professional capability; the availability of additional education and support for midwives; systems offering models for continuity; consistency with local purchasing intentions; and evidence of being able to handle a minimum of 200 deliveries per annum.

- *Systems:* the sites were required to have agreed local *policies* to include professional responsibility and availability; access to the service; referral patterns between professional groups; care from hospital to community. They were required to have *provision* for an available paramedic team or Emergency Obstetric Unit and provision for suitable emergency neonatal resuscitation. They were required to have agreed *protocols* on how care would be managed; communications, including those with the Primary Health Care Team (PHCT); maintenance of records; roles and responsibilities of professionals within the development. They were also required to have *compatible computerised records* and arrangements for the provision of *audit*.

- *Environment:* the sites were required to ensure availability and adequacy of equipment and accommodation and to provide a convenient location for women.

As a result of the tendering exercise, three midwifery group practice (MGP) pilot sites were selected by SETRHA and launched in January 1994, with the intention that they should be funded over a two-year period until December 1995:

1. The Lewisham Maternity Focus at Lewisham Hospital in South London;

2. The JACANES Midwifery Group Practice at the William Harvey Hospital in Ashford, Kent;

3. The South East London Midwifery Group Practice based in Deptford and made up of a group of self-employed midwives operating within the National Health Service (NHS).

The management arrangements for these midwifery group practices are described in more detail in Chapters 2 and 7.

The evaluation

Policy Studies Institute was commissioned to undertake the evaluation of the pilot projects. The research was designed to be both a descriptive study and an evaluation of the effectiveness of the three midwifery group practices. Clinical audit was outside the scope of the PSI evaluation since arrangements for clinical audit were the responsibility of the midwifery group practices themselves (see above). Clinical effectiveness, for example mother and baby morbidity and mortality, was included within the broad areas to be evaluated but only in strictly descriptive terms. Policy Studies Institute was not engaged to be involved in clinical issues or judgements outside the parameters of the expertise of the research team, so that safety issues, for example, could not be fully investigated by the team.

The broad areas to be evaluated were laid down by SETRHA in their brief to the researchers and included:

- comparative costs of the models;
- role clarification of practitioners (obstetrician/midwife/general practitioner);
- access to midwife;
- improvement in the continuity of care and availability of choice for women;
- client satisfaction;
- clinical effectiveness, for example, mother and baby morbidity and mortality.

Criteria against which to evaluate the midwifery group practices were derived from the hypothesis put forward by SETRHA that the pilot sites for the midwifery group practices would provide high quality and cost-effective services to women and their families, who would exhibit increased satisfaction with the service. More specifically SETRHA also set out a number of assumptions upon which the development of the midwifery group practices and the design of the evaluation were based. These assumptions were that:

- Service delivery in a group practice setting would improve continuity of care and carer.
- Direct access to a midwife would be improved if the maternity services were community centred.

- In strengthening the role of midwives in a group practice users would be given greater choice.

- The self-esteem of midwives would be improved, thereby impacting on the quality of care delivered.

- Midwifery group practices would reduce duplication of services to women.

- The roles and responsibilities of practitioners would be clarified.

- Safety would not be reduced.

Methods

The performance of the midwifery group practices was monitored by PSI over an 18-month period (1 April 1994-30 September 1995) using both quantitative and qualitative methods. The range of methods used to collect evidence for the study are summarised below, and more detailed explanation about specific research methods can be found in relevant appendices.

Existing documentation

Information which was necessary to understand the set-up, structure and procedures of the individual midwifery group practices was collected from each of the pilot sites. We reviewed written documents produced by each of the MGPs, including their applications for funding and their protocols.

Monitoring instruments

We designed a common recording system in conjunction with the midwives in the early stages of the evaluation for monitoring the activity, functioning and referral patterns within the three pilot midwifery group practices. The aim was to ensure that a minimum set of common data was collected in all three pilot sites.

(i) Activity/outcome forms

Over the 18-month monitoring period, activity forms were completed by individual midwives to give information about all first consultations and all second and subsequent consultations by the women using the scheme. An outcome form was also completed by the midwife for each woman whose pregnancy had ended by the end of the monitoring period. This system of monitoring was designed to identify the characteristics of users of the pilot projects, the source of their referral to the midwifery group practice, the professionals involved in each consultation, the location of each consultation and the time spent on it, the type and extent of activity involved, and the choices and outcomes for the women at various stages of their pregnancy. The situation was complicated by the fact that all the members of the midwifery group practices were bringing caseloads with them into the monitoring period, made up of women who had booked with the midwives up to five months before April 1994 (see Chapter 3 and Appendix C for further description and discussion of this).

In total 11,742 activity forms were analysed covering the 18-month monitoring period (see Table 3.1) and outcome forms on 1,128 deliveries were analysed for the same period (see Table 3.5). The statistics and findings for each of the midwifery group practices are discussed in Chapters 3 and 4 and in Appendices C and D.

(ii) Diary sheets and duty rota

Midwives were also asked to complete diary sheets over a 2-week period in September 1995 to provide a more in-depth view of the nature and range of activities carried out in their day-to-day work.

Towards the end of the monitoring period we also carried out an analysis of the duty rota for each midwifery group practice over a 5-week period, in order to understand more clearly how duty was organised. The results of both these exercises are reported in Chapter 2 and Appendices A and B.

Interviews

Semi-structured interviews were conducted with midwives, other professionals, and women using the services provided by the midwifery group practices.

(i) MGP midwives

All midwifery group practice midwives were interviewed during May and June 1994 to provide an initial view of their aims and expectations and to identify the criteria against which they themselves would measure their achievements. Where appropriate we also interviewed the senior midwifery managers. The midwives and their managers were also interviewed at the end of the monitoring period to hear of their experiences of the midwifery group practices, the key features of this model of service delivery and to elicit their views on whether or not this model could be replicated elsewhere. We were also interested to find out what factors they felt had affected their performance and success. The views and opinions of the midwives are presented in Chapter 7.

(ii) Other professionals

The pilot midwifery group practice projects were required by SETRHA to clarify the roles and responsibilities of the practitioners involved in the work of the pilot sites. These practitioners included GPs and consultant obstetricians. As part of the evaluation, we interviewed a total of 38 GPs, working within the 'host practices' or locally, both to find out their views on the provision of midwifery and maternity services locally, and more specifically to reflect on the working of the pilot midwifery group practices.

Interviews were conducted with the majority of GPs from the practices participating in the pilots in Lewisham and in Ashford (the 'host practices'), and also with 12 GPs who were based in the vicinity of the Deptford midwifery group practice. We wanted to establish how much they knew about the pilot schemes, the extent and nature of their liaison with the midwives and their assessment of the midwifery group practice as a model of service delivery. We were particularly interested in the perceived strengths and weaknesses of the midwifery group practices in comparison with other working arrangements. We also explored these issues with a small number of consultant obstetricians who were familiar with the pilot midwifery group practices.

The findings from both the GP and consultant obstetrician interviews are presented in Chapter 8.

(iii) Women users of the midwifery group practices

Women using the midwifery group practices were interviewed in order to assess not only their satisfaction with the service, but also their views on the choice of services offered to them by the new model and the extent to which they experienced continuity of care from the same professional.

Semi-structured interviews were conducted with six sample groups of women, drawn randomly from those who booked with the midwifery group practices in April, July and October 1994 and in January, April and July 1995. All the women in these six sample groups were interviewed shortly after they had booked with one of the MGPs. Women in the first four sample groups were also interviewed after they had given birth. (It was not possible to conduct follow-up interviews with most women in the final two sample groups because their expected dates of delivery were outside the monitoring period.)

We conducted interviews with 180 women: a full first interview with 168 women, partial first interviews with 12 women and follow-up interviews with 117 women, giving a total of 297 interviews altogether. Findings from these interviews are presented in Chapters 5 and 6. Sampling and methods are described in detail in Appendix E.

Cost-effectiveness measures

The broad areas to be evaluated by the study included cost-effectiveness measures in order to assess whether the midwifery group practices presented an attractive model of service provision to commissioners and purchasers in terms of both effectiveness and value for money.

At the outset it was unclear how much information would be available from provider units and purchasers on costs and costing mechanisms. It was also clear that some aims of the project would be difficult to measure in cost-effectiveness terms, for example, the intangible benefits of the well-being of mothers.

Interviews were conducted with representatives of the purchasers and providers in each pilot site in order to collect information about contracts, purchasing and funding arrangements. In addition, a range of individuals unconnected with the specific MGPs were consulted for a broader insight into the issues surrounding the costing and purchasing of maternity services.

As we describe more fully in Chapter 9, we found that financial information tended to be crude, fragmented and open to different interpretations and therefore of little practical help in itself to other purchasers and providers in planning midwifery care. We provide cost descriptions for each of the sites to the extent that this was possible, but our main conclusion was that the value of the report is in providing guidance to purchasers and providers on the level and type of resources required to operate and sustain midwifery-led care. These issues are discussed in more detail in Chapters 9 and 10.

Structure and presentation of the report

We should emphasise that this report is essentially an evaluation of three midwifery group practices within their local context. We are aware of the extensive literature on midwifery and maternity services, but, with the agreement of SETRHA, the commissioners of the evaluation, and the steering group set up to oversee the project and the evaluation, we decided from the outset that we would concentrate largely on the empirical data we collected rather than attempt to contextualise it any more than was essential. The report is long and detailed and we considered our approach the most appropriate in the circumstances.

The report structure has been outlined briefly in the preceding description. Chapter 2 and Appendices A and B give a detailed analysis of the aims and organisation of the midwifery group practices. Chapters 3 and 4 and Appendices C and D describe the activity and workload of the midwifery group practices during the antenatal, intrapartum and postnatal period, as well as analysing in detail the characteristics of the users of the services. These three chapters contain a considerable amount of statistical data which may not be of interest to all readers, but are essential background to an understanding of the functioning of the midwifery group practices.

Chapters 5 and 6 describe the women users' experience of antenatal, intrapartum and postnatal care. Chapter 7 looks at the views and experience of the midwives working in the midwifery group practices, and Chapter 8 looks at the views and experience of the GPs and consultant obstetricians concerned. These four chapters contain far less statistical information than the three preceding chapters, but present the findings from the interviews we conducted with key respondents, illustrated by verbatim quotes from the interviews.

Chapter 9 describes and discusses the contracts, purchasing and funding arrangements of the three midwifery group practices and highlights the difficulties in conducting a cost-effectiveness exercise as part of this evaluation. It concentrates on the resource issues involved in operating and sustaining the midwifery group practices in the three pilot sites, in the absence of robust and reliable cost data.

Finally in Chapter 10 we present a detailed discussion of the findings of the evaluation, with the objective of drawing out the lessons which can be learnt from the experience of all those involved in the pilot projects. We explore the implications for policy and practice of the models of working established by the three midwifery group practices. We stress that the aim of the evaluation was not to award prizes but to examine both the successes and failures of the projects in achieving the goals which were set out for them. There are many lessons in this evaluation, not only for those planning midwifery group practices, but for purchasers, providers and planners within the health service in general. We hope that this report will contribute to future debates, not only about maternity services, but will be recognised as having a wider application for other areas of health and social care.

Chapter 2

Aims and organisation of the midwifery group practices

This chapter sets out the aims and objectives of the three midwifery group practices (MGPs) and outlines the way in which care was organised and provided in the three pilot sites. Taking each of the MGPs in turn it highlights key features about the envisaged workload, staffing arrangements and day-to-day activities of the midwives. It provides a context for the more detailed discussion in Chapter 3 of the caseloads of the midwives and their contact with users of the service over the 18-month monitoring period.

Data sources for this chapter include a diary sheet exercise which was completed by all midwives over a 2-week period and, where appropriate, an analysis of the duty rotas over a 5-week period.

The purpose of analysing the duty rotas was to understand more clearly how duty was organised. The aim of asking midwives to fill in diary sheets was to get a clearer picture of how they used their time and the range of activities involved. The findings from this exercise are indicative only, but raise a number of issues for service planning and management which would merit monitoring over the longer term. Tables relating to both exercises are given in Appendix A.

THE LEWISHAM MIDWIFERY GROUP PRACTICE

Aims and objectives
One of the primary objectives of the Lewisham midwifery group practice (known as Lewisham Maternity Focus) was to provide continuity of care and carer from the point of booking with the MGP, through pregnancy, delivery and the postnatal period. It was proposed that women should have increased control over their pregnancy and childbirth and that the new model of care would be more satisfying for women and midwives alike. It was envisaged that midwives would have the opportunity to use and develop their skills and expertise.

The main aims of the MGP as set out in their proposal to SETRHA were:

- to broaden the choice of care and place of delivery offered to Lewisham clients;

- to put the woman first with regard to deciding who provides her care;

- to empower women to make informed choices and to achieve a high quality and standard of maternity care.

Staffing

The Lewisham MGP consisted of 7 full-time midwives who remained in post for the duration of the pilot. Their ages ranged from 27 to 47 years. All but one were married or living with a partner and 4 had children.

Immediately before joining the MGP all 7 midwives were already working in Lewisham. 4 were community midwives (all grade G) and the remainder were hospital midwives (2 at grade F and 1 grade G). The average number of years post-qualification was 15, ranging from 4 to 23 years.

All the members of the MGP were Registered Midwives or State Certified Midwives (SCM) and 2 had higher qualifications in midwifery – either the Diploma in Professional Studies or the Advanced Diploma in Midwifery. Other qualifications held by individual midwives included training in family planning and in parenthood education.

Location of the MGP and access to the service

Facilitating direct access to a midwife was one of SETRHA's aims in setting up the pilot projects with the assumption that access would be improved if the maternity services were community centred.

Location

The Lewisham MGP was community based to ensure ease of access to the service. The 7 midwives had an office base (shared with other community midwives) at Lewisham Hospital, but were attached to 3 local GP practices. These GP practices were selected for the pilot project because they had shown an interest in the pilot and fulfilled the criteria in terms of numbers of women required to ensure that the MGP had an adequate caseload. Some of the community midwives were already established in these GP practices and were familiar with the GPs and the locality, while others were transferred from other practices or from Lewisham Hospital.

The midwives did not visit the office each day but instead received messages or instructions from one of the midwives who was rostered on-call. Midwives who were rostered on-call were responsible for visiting the office to collect any relevant information and to communicate this to colleagues. Weekly group practice meetings were held at one of the 'host' GP practices.

Access to the service

In Lewisham the booking arrangements were initially channelled through the Hospital Antenatal Clinic (ANC). It was envisaged that after a positive pregnancy test women would be referred by their GP to the Hospital ANC where the details of all the women who were registered with the three GP practices taking part in the pilot project would be passed on to the MGP coordinator to arrange booking appointments. This system of referral to the MGP changed very early in the monitoring period to direct referrals from GPs to the MGP. Following the allocation of women to a named midwife, a booking consultation was carried out during which women could choose their preferred options for care during pregnancy and birth.

Direct access to a midwife was a key feature of these schemes and at the first consultation or booking visit with their MGP midwife women were given full details and advice about how and when they should contact their named midwife. In addition to an information leaflet on the MGP, women were given the mobile telephone numbers of both their named midwife, as the first point of contact, and of the other midwives in the MGP. They also received Lewisham Hospital and other central telephone numbers. When midwives were off-duty or otherwise unavailable they diverted their mobile phones to one of the midwives on-call. This meant that women would always have direct access to their named midwife or to another MGP midwife. This was unlike the system in operation in Ashford where mobile phones were not diverted to colleagues working on-call and women had to telephone the JACANES office to find out which midwife was on-call.

Caseload

The proposal for the Lewisham MGP had envisaged 6 midwives undertaking the maternity care of a group of women from a designated geographical patch with a minimum of 200 deliveries per annum. In the event, the patch selected for the pilot project was expected to yield around 240 deliveries per annum and, as described above, it was envisaged that 7 midwives would be needed to carry out this number of deliveries.

The Lewisham MGP was set up to provide midwifery services for women of all risk categories. It did not screen out high risk women because of a concern that this would lead to the provision of a two-tier service. Each woman who was booked by the MGP was assigned a named midwife who would provide all or some of her care in conjunction with other professionals as required throughout her pregnancy. Women of all risk categories had a named midwife, emphasising the one-to-one approach to care which was supported by a group of midwives who could provide the necessary cover if the named midwife was off-duty or otherwise unavailable. It was expected that a substantial proportion of women would choose to have a midwife as their lead professional and would then receive 'midwifery-led' care. A key feature of care was that midwifery involvement would continue if complications arose and the midwife referred the woman to a consultant. If the problem was resolved the midwife could resume lead responsibility.

Protocols

Evidence of clear working practices were required by SETRHA and as part of the study the pilot projects were required to clarify their roles and relationships in relation to other practitioners. Additionally, setting up the MGPs to provide continuity of care and carer posed a number of practical concerns relating to the organisation of work schedules and on-call cover arrangements. In addition to agreeing and making explicit the roles and responsibility of the MGP itself, protocols for working with other professionals and departments were a prerequisite for the provision of a seamless service.

In Lewisham existing protocols were extended to cover the MGP in some instances, and new protocols were introduced where necessary. The following arrangements were in place before the MGP became operational in April 1994:

- *communication document* – this was designed for use by the MGP midwives to inform appropriate professionals about a particular case;
- *casenotes* – were previously carried by women antenatally but this was extended to include the postnatal period also;
- *delivery suite protocol* – was agreed following discussions between obstetricians and midwifery staff at Lewisham. The protocol documentation set out guidelines for the management of patients booked for delivery at the hospital;
- *antenatal care protocol* – set out the types of antenatal care available, visiting schedules, booking visit guidelines, action to take if necessary following the booking visit (referrals to a consultant or GP), and action to take if abnormalities were found or suspected antenatally;
- arrangements for *community obstetric cover;*
- details of the proposed *audit procedures;*
- *communicating with the supervisor of midwives* about untoward events;

- *guidelines for midwifery-led care* – included details of antenatal consultations, making referrals to other professionals, the antenatal visiting schedule, guidelines for labour, birth and the postnatal period. In addition, the document included guidance on the management of antenatal, intrapartum and postnatal emergencies.

Working arrangements

There were a number of important differences between the MGPs in terms of their approach to the organisation of work schedules and on-call arrangements. These reflected some practical differences amongst the MGPs such as their staffing levels, and also variations in the MGP model of care adopted by the different pilot sites.

Lewisham MGP duty rota

In order to determine how duty was organised by the MGP, we carried out an analysis of their duty rota over a 5-week period in August/September 1995. We were particularly interested in the organisation of the regular work schedule and the organisation of on-call cover (see Appendix A).

A flexible work scheduling system was developed by the midwives who took it in turn to organise a monthly duty rota on an internal rotation basis. All staff had the opportunity to make duty requests before the rota was drawn up. A number of key features underpinning the organisation of regular work and on-call cover were identified which included:

- each midwife was scheduled to work 150 hours each month or 37.5 hours each week;

- each midwife worked 2–3 on-calls each week, or 8–11 on-calls each month;

- midwives received 2 days off each week which could be taken together or separately. Midwives were also entitled to 2 weekends off each month.

Continuous cover

Throughout the monitoring period there was a consistent approach to the organisation of care and continuous cover arrangements in Lewisham. Each midwife had responsibility for her own caseload which entailed planning and providing the majority of care and, where possible, attending the woman in labour. The provision of 24-hour cover for all women receiving MGP care was shared by the midwives in the group. Two midwives were rostered on-call each day to provide care for their own clients and cover for colleagues who were off-duty or otherwise unavailable. On-call cover was provided for a 24-hour period beginning at 9 am until 9 am the following morning. Midwives who were on-call simply worked a regular day shift until 5 pm and then continued to provide cover for an additional 16 hours. This 16-hour period will be referred to throughout as residual on-call time.

Having two midwives who were accessible to all women at any point during the day or night was central to achieving continuous cover, but in practice midwives found it difficult to switch off their mobile phones or divert them to colleagues who were on-call because they felt they should be available for women on their own caseloads at all times. The result was that all midwives provided a certain amount of informal out-of-hours cover (when they were off-duty) for women on their own caseload. The midwives usually advised women that they would not divert their mobile phones when off-duty so that they could be contacted if required.

Providing out-of-hours cover to women may have occurred initially because midwives did not feel confident about sharing their workload. In view of the fact that many of the midwives had not worked together before forming the MGP, it may have taken some time before they were comfortable with team cover. However, as a team ethos developed so did midwives' confidence in having colleagues caring for women on their case-loads. The reduction in informal cover in the second year of the monitoring period seems to have resulted from midwives recognising that a group of practitioners working together can achieve more than individuals working alone. In addition, midwives may have recognised that being available for women during scheduled work and on-call time is difficult enough to sustain, without the added pressure of being available when off-duty.

Variations in cover arrangements
Given that midwives worked only 2 weekends each month, not surprisingly, less cover was provided at weekends than during the week. While 2 midwives were scheduled on-call each day from Monday to Friday, only 3 midwives provided on-call cover over the weekend period; 2 working Saturday and 1 Sunday, or vice versa. However, if the weekend was particularly busy, 1 of the 3 midwives provided on-call cover on consecutive days.

Time commitment and flexibility
We used information from both the duty rota analysis and the diary sheets to get a better understanding of the time commitment and flexibility required from midwives under this model of care.

Using the duty rota we looked at the number of regular hours (calculated from the number of day shifts) that the midwives were scheduled to work over the 5 weeks. While some midwives were scheduled to work 5 days (37.5 hours) each week, others were scheduled to work 3, 4 or 6 days, depending on off-duty requests and staff availability for that particular period.

The diary sheets completed by the midwives indicated that while midwives frequently experienced heavy demands on their time both during and outside scheduled work hours, there were also slack periods during scheduled work hours. We found that around 10 per cent of scheduled work time (9 am to 5 pm) was inactive. This slack time can be partly explained by the fact that demands on midwives could not always be predicted. In addition, if on-call midwives were busy during the night they invariably took a few hours to sleep before starting their regular day shift. The amount of 'lost time' over the long term is likely to have implications for the amount of resource required by the model and the sustainability of the service.

In addition to looking at regular work hours we were also interested in the amount of on-call cover that midwives were expected to provide. Having 2 midwives on-call simultaneously meant that the Lewisham MGP provided twice as much on-call cover over the 5 weeks (1,040 hours) as Ashford. The system of cover in Lewisham appeared to be more demanding because of the longer periods of on-call (24 hours on-call rather than day or overnight on-call in Ashford). Even if midwives were not always called upon by clients or colleagues, simply being available obviously limited what they could do socially during this time. Individual midwives provided between 96 and 192 hours of on-call cover (6–12 on-calls) over the 5-week period.

Looking at the number of regular work hours and on-call hours together gives a good picture of the degree of commitment required of midwives on a continuous basis. We therefore established the amount of time midwives were scheduled to work and provide on-call cover between one day off and the next. We have already seen that midwives were generally scheduled to work 37.5 hours each week (excluding any on-call work). However, if a day off was taken at the beginning of one week and the next day off was half way through or at the end of the following week, midwives had to work lengthy periods between days off.

Table A.1 (Appendix A) shows the longest number of day shifts (9 am to 5 pm in the evening) and residual on-call hours that midwives were scheduled to work between days off. The table indicates that 4 of the 7 midwives were scheduled to work as many as 8 consecutive day shifts and 3 of those midwives were scheduled to provide on-call cover (an additional 16 hours) every second day. Another midwife was scheduled to work 10 regular day shifts and provide on-call cover on every second day.

Day-to-day activities

Given that a major objective of the evaluation was to establish whether the MGP model as developed in these pilot sites could be replicated elsewhere, it was important to understand how resources had been used. In this context the two-week diary sheet exercise was used to indicate how much time had been spent by midwives on different activities.

Table A.2 shows the amount of time recorded by midwives across a range of activities. The final two columns on the table show the number of hours that midwives were scheduled to work from their duty rota (regular day shift time only), and the actual amount of time that was recorded by the midwives during the 2-week exercise. We were also able to identify whether activities occurred in regular hours, on-call time or out-of-hours. During this 2-week period nearly 20 per cent of the time attributed to activities by midwives was during periods of on-call. Another 13 per cent of time recorded on activities was out-of-hours.

Direct care activities

We asked midwives to record their time under direct care and a range of other activities. Direct care was primarily direct contact with the women and included booking consultations, subsequent antenatal consultations (also referred to as second and subsequent consultations), intrapartum care, postnatal consultations, specialist appointments and classes. Over half of all time recorded was spent on direct care (55 per cent). Table A.3 shows the amount of time spent by midwives on each of the direct care activities.

Although the average amount of time spent by a midwife on direct care was around 52 hours, the actual time recorded by individual midwives ranged from 31 to 72 hours over the 2-week period. The differences are clearly due to the varying demands on midwives' time, which seems to have been related in particular to the provision of intrapartum care during this period. While postnatal and antenatal care (first and subsequent consultations) accounted for a substantial proportion of time recorded on direct care overall, busy periods invariably resulted from attending women in labour.

We found that in total the Lewisham MGP carried out more second and subsequent antenatal consultations and more postnatal consultations than elsewhere. However, in so doing the midwives spent on average 24 per cent *less time* on second and subsequent antenatal consultations and 16 per cent *less time* on postnatal consultations than midwives in Ashford.

The small amount of time recorded on classes is attributed to the fact that some of the midwives did not hold classes in September.

Other activities

While direct care activities are the core of the MGP's overall work, other activities are essential to the effective functioning of the MGP. In order to make an informed judgement on the sustainability of the model of MGP care it is important to look at care provision against a whole host of activities indirectly related to caring for women. Table A.2 indicates the amount of time spent by each midwife on these other activities and the total MGP time for each activity or category of activities.

Administrative tasks were the most time-consuming activity after direct care activities, accounting for 14 per cent of all time recorded. Lewisham and Ashford MGPs spent roughly the same proportion of time on administrative activities and this was greater than the proportion of time spent in Deptford. Table A.2 shows that the average time spent on administrative tasks was 13 hours, ranging for individual midwives from 4.5 to 22 hours.

Miscellaneous tasks which accounted for 6 per cent of all recorded time included such activities as collecting and restocking equipment and supplies, preparing booking packs, attending a fire lecture, giving a lecture/talk on the MGP. Two midwives who had responsibility for team coordination and client allocation spent around a third of their recorded time on administrative and miscellaneous activities alone. It is important to recognise that any extra tasks carried out by midwives to ensure the smooth running of the MGP could be time-consuming and were often carried out when the midwives were off-duty.

Travel accounted for 13 per cent of the time recorded by the midwives. Roughly the same proportion of time was spent on travel in Lewisham and Deptford and this was slightly higher than in Ashford. This may be due to the fact that both of these MGPs carried out the majority of their consultations in the client's home. Table A.2 indicates that the amount of time recorded by individual midwives ranged from 4.5 to 22.5 hours. It is possible that travel time was under-recorded by some midwives but there also appears to be a link between the time spent on travel and intrapartum care, as some midwives who spent more time on intrapartum care recorded less time on travel.

7 per cent of all recorded time in Lewisham was spent on meetings which was lower than elsewhere. Over half the time recorded was spent on midwives' meetings and the remainder on other meetings. Table A.2 shows that the time recorded by individual midwives varied widely and that midwives who spent the most time on intrapartum care usually recorded less time on meetings.

A relatively small proportion of time was spent on telephone calls (5 per cent of all recorded time). Both Ashford and Deptford MGPs spent a higher proportion of time on telephone calls. Over half of the time recorded in Lewisham was attributed to calls made to or taken from clients. Nearly a third of the time was spent on calls to other MGP midwives while the remainder of the time was spent on miscellaneous calls. Table A.2 indicates that the average time spent on telephone calls for each midwife during the exercise was 5 hours, but the actual time spent by individual midwives ranged from 2 to 8.5 hours.

THE JACANES MIDWIFERY GROUP PRACTICE

Aims and objectives of the MGP

The proposal for the JACANES MGP in Ashford to take part in the evaluation was put forward by a group of enthusiastic community midwives and their managers who sought to maximise the skills of the midwife, and to reduce duplication of professional roles when caring for mothers. It was their view that women should feature strongly in the planning of their care for pregnancy and birth and that they should have the option of receiving midwifery-led care based in the community. The main aims set out in the JACANES proposal were that women should:

• be given unbiased information to inform their choice of place of delivery;

• have increased control and participation in their care;

• be involved in selecting a lead professional who would provide continuity of care and carer;

• be attended by one midwife in labour, as set out in the Short Report, 1980.

Staffing

The MGP originally consisted of 6 midwives, 5 of whom worked full-time and 1 part-time. One midwife went on maternity leave 6 months into the monitoring period and was replaced by another full-time midwife. On returning from maternity leave in September 1995 she organised a job share with 1 of the midwives within the MGP. Also in September 1995 1 of the midwives reduced her hours, leaving the MGP with 3 part-time midwives and 4 full-time midwives – 5 grade G and 2 grade F – (a whole-time equivalent of 6 midwives).

Immediately before joining the MGP all 7 midwives involved were working in the Ashford area. Four were community midwives (all grade G) and 3 were hospital midwives (2 grade E and 1 grade F). On joining the MGP, the 2 grade E midwives were upgraded to grade F. The number of years post-qualification ranged from 5 to 22 years.

The age profile of midwives in JACANES was similar to Lewisham, ranging from 30 to 49 years. All were married and all had children.

All were Registered Midwives (or SCM) and 2 held higher qualifications in midwifery – the Diploma in Professional Studies in Midwifery, or the Advanced Diploma in Midwifery.

Location of the MGP and access to the service

Location

This MGP was set up to serve a large semi-rural area (120 square miles) and at the outset it was decided that the MGP midwives would remain GP based where suitable accommodation was available. Five GP practices were selected as 'host' practices in Ashford, Willesborough, Wye and Charing. As in Lewisham, some of the MGP midwives who had previously been community midwives were already established in the GP practices and were therefore familiar with the GPs and the locality. The ex-hospital midwives who joined the MGP were transferred to the remaining 'host' practices.

Although the service was to be community based, it was decided that the MGP midwives should have an office at the William Harvey Hospital in Ashford to ensure adequate administrative support and sufficient space for the necessary office equipment. The office also provided a central meeting place for all the MGP midwives who were attached to the dispersed GP practices. Team meetings, however, were often held in a midwife's home, both because of limited office space and for the convenience of midwives who might otherwise have to travel to the hospital on a day off.

A community hall in Ashford was identified as the most accessible venue in which to hold a monthly drop-in service (similar to Meet and Greet sessions in Lewisham). This service was run in rotation by the midwives themselves.

Access to the service

Booking arrangements for the service were arranged primarily through GP practices. It was envisaged that women would be referred by their GP to the MGP to arrange a booking consultation following a positive pregnancy test. Alternatively, if the woman went directly to the MGP, the midwife would inform the GP of this by letter, stating that a booking consultation would be arranged following a positive test result. The midwife forwarded a referral form to the hospital to book a maternity bed if this was the woman's chosen place of birth. Women who required consultant care were referred to the hospital to arrange further care.

Protocol 9 (see below) specified the arrangements for ensuring that women had continuous access either to their named midwife, or another MGP midwife. Women were advised at the booking consultation to use their named midwife's mobile phone number as their first point of contact. If the mobile telephone was switched off or the midwife was not contactable, they were advised to contact the main telephone number of the MGP office at William Harvey Hospital, where they were informed of the mobile telephone number of the midwife who was on-call.

Caseload

The JACANES MGP proposed that it would provide midwifery services for a combined caseload of up to 500 women of all risk categories. Of this total the MGP envisaged providing continuity of care and carer for around 200 women with uncomplicated pregnancies for an entire episode of care, including delivery. These women had the option of choosing midwifery-led care and having a midwife as lead professional. The MGP midwives also envisaged providing some antenatal and postnatal care to women with complicated pregnancies, working in conjunction with the lead professional who might be a consultant obstetrician or GP, but not providing intrapartum care for this group of women.

The size of the envisaged caseload for individual midwives differed according to their grade. The G grade midwives were seen as principal care providers with a caseload of 40 women, compared to F grade associate midwives who were expected to carry a reduced caseload of 24 women. These projected caseload figures were based on the 200 or so women booked for a full episode of care. They did not take into account the 290 or so high risk women for whom the midwives could potentially provide some antenatal and postnatal care.

In practice, providing care for women of all risk groups posed a number of problems for JACANES, especially in relation to the midwives' workload. This was partly because a large proportion of high risk women requested DOMINO (Domiciliary In and Out) deliveries which required more antenatal input from the MGP midwives than originally anticipated and in addition involved the midwives in intrapartum care. Providing intrapartum care for this group of women was not discussed in the proposal nor taken into account in the original staffing plans for the MGP.

Another factor contributing to the increase in workload was that midwives themselves found it increasingly difficult to decline requests for shared care (with greater input from JACANES MGP midwives) especially if the midwives had looked after some of the women in previous pregnancies. Midwives were also concerned that if they did not provide the same choices for pregnancy and birth to women of all risk groups they would create a two-tier system of care which would favour the low risk group of women in terms of choice and continuity.

It became increasingly apparent that high risk women were receiving more care than the infrastructure of the MGP was capable of providing. At the same time women with uncomplicated pregnancies, who went post term, were at risk of being transferred to the hospital teams and not being attended by their MGP midwife at the delivery. It was clear that midwives could not sustain a double caseload if the aims of the pilot were to be achieved and women with uncomplicated pregnancies were to receive continuity of care and carer for the full episode of care including delivery. The problem was exacerbated by the fact that the overall caseload for the MGP was nearer to 600 than the projected 500.

In order to address these workload issues the Trust secured funds from East Kent Health Authority to employ an additional six midwives to staff a second MGP. Called JACANES II, this MGP was responsible from March 1995 for providing care to high risk women. At that point approximately 80 women who were deemed high risk were transferred from JACANES I into JACANES II and were no longer included in the pilot evaluation. After March 1995 all women were assessed to determine risk before their booking consultation and were then signposted to JACANES I or JACANES II for future care.

Protocols

In JACANES, as in Lewisham, an extensive number of protocols were drawn up by the midwives in conjunction with their midwifery services manager before the MGP became operational. These are outlined below:

- *Protocol 1: communication systems between hospital staff and the MGP* – gave guidance on how to contact MGP midwives;

- *Protocol 2: selecting a mother for MGP care* – listed complications which excluded a woman from MGP care – thus acting as eligibility criteria for obstetrician-led care;

- *Protocol 3: antenatal booking* – provided guidelines on the booking consultation, information to be made available to women and action to take on key areas;

- *Protocol 4: referral of women when an uncomplicated pregnancy becomes complicated* – listed conditions of the baby/mother which should trigger a referral to a Consultant Obstetrician for an opinion and possible transfer of care;

- *Protocol 5: neonatal transfer from hospital to the community* – provided guidelines on the transfer policy for babies delivered to MGP mothers who wished to go home from hospital within 24 hours of having an uncomplicated delivery;

- *Protocol 6: transfer of mother from hospital to community* – set out the transfer policy for mothers with an uncomplicated pregnancy and delivery who wished to go home from hospital within 6–24 hours after delivery;

- *Protocol 7: antenatal referral for emergency admission* – outlined action to be taken by the midwife when specific complications arose;

- *Protocol 8: care of mother in labour* – gave guidelines on the role and responsibilities of the MGP midwife in caring for a woman in labour;

- *Protocol 9: contacting MGP midwives* – outlined how a woman could contact her named midwife or another MGP midwife;

- *Protocol 10: the role of the liaison midwife* – outlined the role of the liaison midwife in collecting the details of all mothers before they were transferred home, and the organisation of initial postnatal home visits by the MGP midwives;

- *Protocol 11: safety* – set out guidelines for the MGP midwives on handing over duties following a busy period of overnight on-call, and guidelines on taking and requesting time owing.

Working arrangements

The different approaches adopted to the organisation of work and on-call cover enables us to identify certain criteria that are likely to contribute to sustainable practice and replicability in each location.

JACANES duty rota

In order to look at the working arrangements adopted in Ashford we carried out an analysis of the duty rota for a 5-week period in August/September 1995.

A semi-flexible work scheduling system was developed by this MGP which provided individual midwives with the opportunity to indicate particular duty or time-off preferences. The MGP also took responsibility for drawing up their own duty rota and this was carried out on a monthly basis by midwives in rotation. The key features underpinning the organisation of regular work and on-call cover were:

- each full-time midwife was rostered for up to 12 on-calls (all clients) each month, and part-time staff provided less on-call cover;

- midwives received 2 days off each week and frequently opted for set days off (often 1 day one week and 3 the next), taking into account both the need to cover their own clinics during the week and individual preferences. A similar arrangement existed for part-time midwives;

- midwives had every second weekend off;

- full-time midwives took 1 extra day off each month to compensate for the longer length of the regular day shift in operation (9 hours).

Continuous cover

As in Lewisham, the key to scheduling work and organising cover was to ensure that a midwife was available for all clients at any point of the day or night. A regular day shift from 8 am until 5 pm was introduced at the outset. Each midwife had responsibility for her own caseload but, unlike Lewisham, midwives in Ashford were largely responsible for providing care and continuous cover for women on their own caseload. Within the first few months of operation midwives found that this arrangement was not sustainable given the volume of work associated with holding 'double caseloads'.

Other options for ensuring 24-hour cover were subsequently investigated and the preferred solutions identified by the midwives were to supplement single caseload cover with a more extensive team cover arrangement, and to split 24-hour cover into day and night cover. The MGP subsequently operated day and overnight cover for all clients alongside a third on-call arrangement whereby midwives provided cover for women on their own caseloads (see Appendix B for full details of cover arrangements).

Variations in cover arrangements

One of the major differences between the on-call arrangements in Ashford and Lewisham was that 2 midwives provided 24-hour on-call cover simultaneously in Lewisham, whereas in Ashford 1 midwife provided on-call cover during the day and another midwife provided on-call cover overnight. Given the MGP's staffing levels, having 2 midwives on-call simultaneously would not have been possible. Although midwives were scheduled to provide up to 12 on-calls each month in Ashford this was less demanding than in Lewisham where midwives provided up to eleven 24-hour on-calls each month.

In seeking a balance between providing continuous cover to women receiving MGP care and ensuring equitable and sustainable working arrangements, each midwife was entitled to every second weekend off. A predictable result was that the number of midwives scheduled to work or provide on-call cover on weekdays was greater than at weekends. On a typical weekday, staff cover consisted of 1 on-call midwife and at least 1–2 other midwives who were scheduled to work a regular day shift. In contrast, the weekend period was often staffed by on-call midwives only. On some occasions 1 midwife was scheduled to work a regular day shift on Saturday and/or Sunday. It must be noted however that the analysis of the duty rota took place when some of the midwives were on annual leave, and limited staff availability invariably resulted in reduced cover.

Time commitment and flexibility

Differences between Lewisham and Ashford MGPs in relation to the number of hours that midwives were scheduled to work resulted mainly from the fact that all the midwives in Lewisham were full-time, whereas part-time midwives featured more in Ashford.

Scheduled work hours for each JACANES midwife varied from week to week depending on whether they were full-time or part-time, and the staff availability at that particular time. Midwives were scheduled to work 2–6 days each week. We have already seen that the level of activity in

Lewisham tended to fluctuate and this was also the case in Ashford. Busy periods resulted in midwives working over and above the scheduled number of hours (i.e. when they were not officially on duty), and slack periods resulted in midwives working less than their scheduled hours. As a result, time owing was often taken during the slack periods. The diary sheets revealed a similar proportion of inactive scheduled work time for Lewisham and Ashford (10 per cent) over the 2-week period.

As with Lewisham, we explored the number of additional hours that were required from JACANES midwives in providing day and night time cover. Our analysis shows that this MGP was scheduled to provide around half the number of on-call hours (548.5 hours) provided by the Lewisham MGP. The amount of cover provided by individual midwives depended on whether they were working full-time or part-time.

The time that individual midwives spent in providing own caseload cover is difficult to calculate because of the flexible nature of this on-call cover arrangement. However, the duty rota analysis suggests that over the 5-week period the midwives could have provided in total an additional 200 hours of own caseload cover.

We looked at the longest number of scheduled work and on-call cover hours for each midwife between one day off and the next. Table A.4 shows both scheduled hours and residual on-call hours. It is interesting to note that the highest number of continuous hours calculated for a midwife in Ashford was 78 hours while the lowest number of hours for a midwife in Lewisham was 69.5 hours. The time involved in providing own caseload cover has not been taken into account in this analysis, but obviously this places even more demands on the midwives' time.

As this MGP consisted of full-time and part-time midwives flexibility was paramount. One example of the extra demands made on midwives was that in order to ensure that part-time midwives provided their quota of on-call cover, they occasionally provided on-call cover before a day off.

Day-to-day activities

Midwives in Ashford, like those in Lewisham, completed diary sheets accounting for all their time spent on activities during a 2-week period in September/October 1995. Table A.5 shows the amount of time recorded by midwives across a range of activities. We were able to identify whether these activities took place in regular hours, on-call hours or out-of-hours. We found that nearly 13 per cent of activities were reported during on-call periods and 20 per cent were recorded as out-of-hours.

Direct care activities

For the purposes of the diary sheet exercise, direct care activities in Ashford covered the same range of contact with the women as in

Lewisham. On this basis we found that the Ashford MGP spent a smaller proportion of recorded time overall on direct care activities (less than 50 per cent) than in Lewisham or Deptford.

The average time spent by JACANES midwives on direct care was 32 hours but, as Table A.6 illustrates, the actual time recorded by individual midwives varied from 13.5 to 46 hours. Looking at individual direct care activities it is possible to see that, for intrapartum care alone, only 2 midwives spent any significant time on this activity during the 2-week period. Overall, intrapartum care accounted for only 11 per cent of all time recorded.

Nearly one fifth of all recorded time was attributed to antenatal care i.e. first and subsequent consultations. 11 per cent of recorded time was attributed to carrying out postnatal consultations. Midwives spent, on average, more time than Lewisham on both subsequent antenatal and postnatal consultations over the 2-week diary period. However, as we demonstrate in Chapter 3, this did not hold for the full 18-month monitoring period during which JACANES midwives spent the least time on second and subsequent consultations.

While only a small proportion of time overall was spent on classes it is important to note that three-quarters of this time recorded by midwives was during out-of-hours time. This supports reports from the midwives and their manager that classes were largely provided during their own time. Very little time was recorded on specialist consultations by midwives during the 2-week period.

Other activities

Table A.5 shows the amount of time spent by midwives and the MGP in total on all other activities indirectly related to caring for women. A slightly higher proportion of time was spent on telephone calls in Ashford (6 per cent) than in Lewisham (5 per cent) compared with Deptford (11 per cent). Roughly the same amount of time was spent making or receiving calls to/from clients, and in calling other MGP midwives. Table A.5 shows that the average time midwives spent on telephone calls during the two weeks was around 5 hours, but that the time individual midwives spent on the telephone ranged from as little as 2 hours up to almost 9 hours.

12 per cent of all recorded time was attributed to meetings. The relatively high figure recorded on team meetings compared to Lewisham arises from the fact that most of the JACANES midwives were able to attend team meetings, whereas in Lewisham attendance was reduced by the demands of on-call. Around one fifth of all time spent on meetings in Ashford was recorded during out-of-hours time, reinforcing a concern expressed by some JACANES midwives about attending meetings on their days off.

Even though it covered a large rural area, this MGP reported a slightly lower proportion of overall time on travel (11 per cent) than Lewisham (13 per cent) and Deptford (14 per cent). A factor here is that most ante-natal consultations in Ashford were held at the GP practices, rather than at the women's homes, thus reducing the amount of travelling by midwives. In contrast, antenatal consultations in Lewisham and Deptford were main-ly held in the women's homes, which would require more travelling.

More time (15 per cent) was recorded by JACANES midwives on administrative tasks than any other activity outside direct care. Table A.5 shows that the average time spent by each midwife on administrative activ-ities was 11 hours and the time spent by individual midwives ranged from 6 to 14.5 hours. It is important to note that some of the administrative tasks recorded by midwives in Lewisham and Ashford were carried out by the practice manager in Deptford.

Around 11 per cent of time recorded by JACANES midwives was spent on a range of miscellaneous activities and much of this was out-of-hours time. Almost half of the time spent on miscellaneous tasks was attributed to one midwife who prepared a proposal for the Kent Business Awards. Other activities included liaison work, restocking equipment, and giving a talk on the MGP.

DEPTFORD MIDWIFERY GROUP PRACTICE

Aims and objectives of the MGP

The proposal submitted by the group of midwives in Deptford was to establish a self-managed midwifery group practice within the NHS which would secure funding from the local health authorities. At the time of sub-mitting their bid the group were already in the process of seeking funding from South East London Health Authority (subsequently Lambeth Southwark and Lewisham Health Commission) and Greenwich and Bexley Health Authority. The proposal suggested that the MGP could provide the high quality care envisaged both in *Changing Childbirth* (1993) and the House of Commons Health Select Committee Report on Maternity Services (1992).

The main objectives set out in their proposal were:

• to prepare women for labour, birth and the care and feeding of her child which would include informing women and their partners about the choices open to them;

• to ensure safe care by referring women to other professionals, when appropriate, and to achieve positive outcomes in the birth of mature, live and healthy infants;

- to foster equal responsibility between the woman and midwife, and encourage women to evaluate their care;

- to provide continuity of care through a partnership of two named midwives caring for the woman throughout pregnancy, labour and up to 28 days postnatally;

- to ensure that the birth of the baby is as emotionally satisfying as possible and a pleasurable experience for the whole family.

Staffing

The bid put forward to SETRHA suggested that the Deptford MGP would be a self-managing partnership of 6 midwives. The proposal also stated that the midwives would be self-employed and therefore would have responsibility for managing their own tax, national insurance, pension and personal liability insurance. Details of these arrangements, including the pay and grading equivalents adopted by the MGP, are included in Chapter 9.

When the MGP became operational there were, in fact, 7 midwives in place, 6 full-time and 1 part-time. They were supported by a part-time practice manager who, during the monitoring period, increasingly took on the role of health resource worker and the MGP recruited a new part-time practice manager. The age range of the 7 Deptford midwives was very similar to Lewisham and JACANES. Five of the midwives were married and two were living as married. Five of the 7 had children.

The background of the midwives in the Deptford MGP was more varied than in the other two MGPs. Immediately before the MGP started operating within the NHS three of the seven midwives had worked from home as independent midwives, one had worked as a bank midwife, two had worked in hospital midwifery in other parts of London and one had been a community midwife. Of the four midwives who had previously worked within the NHS, two had been on grade E, one grade F and the other grade G. While all but one had gained experience of hospital midwifery post-qualification, three had not previously worked as community midwives. The number of years experience post-qualification ranged from less than 1 to 21 years. The original practice manager, who also acted as the health resource worker, was an approved mental health social worker.

This MGP experienced considerable staff turnover compared to the other two groups. Because of funding uncertainties, which cast the future of the practice in doubt, and difficulties in maintaining staff relations, 3 midwives left the MGP in March and April 1995. One midwife returned to independent practice, one took up a midwifery management post and another took up a post as a community midwife. A new midwife was recruited to a part-time post in the MGP in May 1995.

Location of the MGP and access to the service

Location

Given that one of the eligibility criteria for the service was that it should serve local women, especially those living in council accommodation, the MGP midwives decided to base themselves in rented offices at a Community Centre in Deptford. The premises were acquired to provide suitable space for a walk-in shopfront/information centre and a library service for local women. It was envisaged that pregnancy testing and pregnancy counselling services would be carried out there, in addition to providing antenatal and postnatal groups, antenatal consultations and office administration. The original office space proved unsuitable for all these tasks and activities and the midwives moved to a larger suite of rooms within the same building in April 1995.

Access

It was envisaged that women would either refer themselves to the Deptford MGP, or be referred by other professionals such as local GPs, consultant obstetricians or other midwives. The group ran a number of local antenatal and postnatal classes free of charge to all women, even if they were not receiving midwifery care from the MGP. This facility, combined with the free pregnancy testing service and the proposed shopfront premises, were identified as important routes for attracting bookings to the core midwifery service.

One of the potential drawbacks for the Deptford MGP in terms of attracting referrals was the fact that the practice had to generate the business itself. Unlike the other two pilot sites, where midwives were based in GP practices and had a guaranteed client source, the MGP in Deptford did not have the same opportunities to ensure a steady stream of referrals.

Caseload

The Deptford midwives proposed that they would undertake the midwifery care of 200 women per annum. The midwives envisaged working in three partnerships, with each partnership responsible for the entire midwifery care of up to 66 women. They aimed to target certain groups of women who satisfied eligibility criteria for special needs which were set out in their service contract with purchasers. These contract conditions and their implications for funding are fully discussed in Chapter 9. The MGP also intended to operate as a health resource for local women who would not necessarily be in receipt of midwifery services.

A complication in Deptford, which had implications both for the operation of the MGP and for the evaluation, was that before the MGP became a pilot site the midwives were already caring for a group of some 30 women, many of whom had booked as self-financing clients, and some 40 women who had booked elsewhere before 1 April 1994. These 70 women continued to receive care from the midwives once the pilot started and the MGP transferred some of the funding from the local health authorities, which was intended for new clients booked after 1 April 1994, to cover the cost of providing the service to this existing group of women. The implications of this are discussed in Chapter 9.

Protocols
A number of protocols were requested by SETRHA from all the MGPs and included:

- guidelines setting out how the MGP would promote, manage and achieve its objectives through inter-agency working;
- evidence of communication documents designed for liaison with other professionals;
- guidelines on managing emergencies;
- details of audit procedures;
- documentation on safety issues;
- plans for staff education and support.

Although some of these issues were addressed in their business plan and in their contracts with purchasers, the Deptford midwives, unlike the other two MGPs, did not provide detailed protocols. In response to SETRHA's request the MGP stated that their approach was to practise within the context of the Midwives' Rules and the Midwife's Code of Practice, and with the support of the local supervisor of midwives. In emergencies they stated that they would refer directly to the senior obstetrician and/or paediatrician on-call and would access the relevant emergency services.

Working arrangements
We have already highlighted some of the distinguishing features of the Deptford MGP model. Another difference was that, unlike Lewisham and Ashford, the Deptford MGP did not have a duty rota as such, but it was still possible to identify key features in the organisation of work and continuous cover. These included:

- Midwives worked in mixed partnerships within which one took on the role of primary named midwife, and the other the role of secondary named midwife. The primary midwife was usually seen as the first point of contact and women had the mobile telephone numbers of both midwives in the partnership and the MGP office. Phone numbers of other midwives in the MGP were also made available to women at the first consultation or booking visit.

- Midwives were available to meet the needs of women and provide support to colleagues on a continuous 24-hour basis. This arrangement had an inherent flexibility which enabled midwives to organise their own work.

- Midwives did not have scheduled time-off apart from blocks of annual leave taken throughout the year.

- Clients were allocated to partnerships according to their expected date of delivery and midwives' annual leave arrangements.

- Because all midwives within the MGP were available on a continuous 24-hour basis, the most notable difference between full-time and part-time midwives working within the group was in the size of their caseloads.

- Full-time midwives booked four women each month as a primary midwife and another four women as a secondary midwife, while part-time midwives booked two women each month as a primary midwife and two women as a secondary midwife.

Continuous cover

The organisation of care and continuous 24-hour cover which was agreed by the midwives mirrored the caseload practice approach, whereby each midwife took ultimate responsibility for the care and cover arrangements for women on her own caseload. Women booked with partnerships according to their expected date of delivery and taking into account midwives' availability and annual leave arrangements.

The partnership arrangement was pivotal to the organisation and provision of care. Initially the midwives worked in fixed partnerships, but this was modified some months into the pilot because the midwives found that mixed partnerships – whereby midwives did not always work in the same pair – facilitated a more flexible approach. While responsibility for providing both care and cover for women booked with the MGP lay primarily with the various partnerships, other midwives in the group also provided back-up and support when required.

The provision of 24-hour cover by each of the midwives on a continuous basis, rather than by a limited number of midwives on an intermittent basis, was a distinguishing feature of the MGP model adopted in Deptford. In contrast, the Ashford MGP operated a combination of on-call cover for their own caseloads and on-call cover for all women. The Lewisham MGP introduced shared cover from the outset, with on-call midwives available to all women being cared for by the MGP, thus leaning much more towards a team midwifery approach, especially for continuous cover. However, in practice it must be recognised that initially the Lewisham MGP midwives also provided 'informal' out-of-hours cover for women on their own caseloads by not diverting their mobile phones to the on-call midwife.

Providing 24-hour continuous cover may have given the Deptford midwives the independence of organising their work according to the particular demands of their own caseloads, but the down side of this approach was that midwives did not have scheduled time off apart from annual leave. We have already seen that in the other MGPs, and particularly in Lewisham where midwives provided 24-hour on-call cover quite frequently, not being called upon when providing on-call cover did not compensate for the fact that midwives had to be available for clients and colleagues for fixed periods of time. We discuss in Chapter 7 what midwives themselves thought of their working arrangements and the demands these placed upon their work and home lives.

The partnership approach adopted in Deptford may have benefits for women being cared for by the MGP because they get to know and often see both midwives during pregnancy, and may be attended by one or both midwives at delivery. However, in terms of potential replication of the model, fixed or mixed partnerships arrangements may also introduce a level of inflexibility and time commitment from midwives which may make the model unattractive to managers and midwives alike.

Day-to-day activities

As in Lewisham and Ashford, the Deptford midwives completed diary sheets over a 2-week period. In order to determine the take-up of midwives' time, they were asked to record activities in a similar manner to the other MGPs. For instance, activities carried out between 9 am to 5 pm were recorded under 'regular work hours'. Other activities carried out after this time were recorded 'outside regular hours' – from 5 pm until 9 am.

Table A.7 shows that the MGP recorded 480 hours on day-to-day activities during the 2-week period and around a quarter of this time was recorded outside regular hours. Not surprisingly, the demands on midwives' time fluctuated over the 2-week period. Full-time midwives recorded more time on various activities than their part-time colleagues but even so there were significant demands on the part-timers, with one recording 82 hours and the other 56 hours, over the 2-week period.

In Deptford, having all midwives providing 24-hour continuous cover ensured that women had direct access to their primary and/or secondary midwife at all times, but it invariably led to lengthy periods of inactivity and redundant time. For example, over the 2-week period one of the part-time midwives was inactive (recording around 2 hours or less on activities) for around half of the overall exercise.

Direct care activities

Although the Deptford midwives were available on a 24-hour basis similar patterns of activity could be seen across the MGPs. Table A.8 indicates that direct care activities accounted for over half of all time recorded for the MGP. While the amount of time spent by individual midwives on direct care varied, the average per midwife was 51 hours over the 2-week period.

Of the total time recorded on direct care, roughly the same proportions were spent on antenatal, and postnatal consultations by the MGP. It was particularly interesting that the Deptford midwives spent more time with women than Lewisham or JACANES midwives at both antenatal and post-natal consultations. This finding is reinforced in Chapter 3 where we demonstrate that throughout the 18-month monitoring period the Deptford MGP consistently spent more time on consultations with women than the other MGPs.

Providing intrapartum care was the most time-consuming of all the direct care activities in Deptford and between a quarter and a third of the time recorded was outside regular hours. While midwives spent on average 14 hours on intrapartum care over the 2-week period, invariably some midwives spent more time than others attending women at birth. Again this was attributable to the particular demands on an individual midwife's time during the 2-week period in question, and not necessarily a result of working full-time or part-time.

Information recorded on the diary sheets suggests that midwives in Deptford were more likely to accompany women to specialist appointments than midwives in Lewisham or in Ashford and, as highlighted in Chapter 3, this is borne out by the completed activity sheets over the 18-month monitoring period. What is interesting is that three-quarters of the time recorded on specialist appointments was outside regular hours.

All the midwives reported spending time on classes, but this sometimes related to National Childbirth Trust (NCT) rather than MGP classes.

Other activities

The distribution of time spent on a variety of support activities which were indirectly related to caring for women is shown in Table A.7.

Travel was the most time-consuming activity outside direct care, accounting for 14 per cent of all time recorded by midwives. Nearly a quarter of this time was recorded outside regular hours. Midwives in Deptford spent a similar proportion of time on travel to the Lewisham midwives and a slightly higher proportion than the Ashford midwives.

Telephone calls accounted for a greater proportion of the time recorded by the Deptford MGP than elsewhere (11 per cent of all recorded time) with around one third of this outside regular hours. More time was spent on calls to clients than on calls to other MGP midwives.

Attending meetings, particularly MGP meetings, appeared time-consuming with roughly the same proportion of time recorded on meetings as on telephone calls (11 per cent of recorded time).

Much less time was spent on administrative tasks by the midwives in Deptford than in Lewisham or Ashford, possibly due to the role of the practice manager in the day-to-day operation of the MGP. It is notable that some of the tasks associated with the MGP's contractual arrangements, such as report writing and attending monitoring meetings with purchasers, were a feature of this MGP's day-to-day activities that did not arise for the other MGPs where contractual negotiations were conducted more centrally.

Miscellaneous activities, which accounted for a small proportion of the overall time recorded by the midwives, included giving a lecture, teaching student midwives, attending study day activities, taking blood samples to the laboratory and preparing for an advisory group meeting. One of the midwives recorded that she had provided childcare for a client's child who had to be admitted as an emergency to hospital. This is significant because during discussions with the midwives they reported providing a high degree of social support to some of the women receiving MGP care. This type of support did not feature in diary sheets elsewhere.

Chapter 3

Activity and workload of the midwifery group practices

One of the primary objectives of setting up the midwifery group practices (MGPs) was to provide 'woman centred care'. A key feature of this form of care is said to be that it provides increased options and choices for women and the opportunity to make informed decisions about issues such as choice of carer in pregnancy and at birth, and choice of location of birth. Another important feature of such care is accessibility and familiarity. The MGPs were set up as small groups of midwives working together to provide community-based care. Each woman could get to know a named midwife from the group who would provide most of her care during pregnancy and, if possible, attend her in labour.

The first part of this chapter looks at the workload and activity of the MGPs over the monitoring period from 1 April 1994 to 30 September 1995. The second part of the chapter looks at the numbers and characteristics of the service users who booked their care with the MGPs, their preferences for care in pregnancy and childbirth and the extent to which those preferences differed from the actual care they received. It discusses in detail their antenatal care. Intrapartum and postnatal care are discussed in Chapter 4.

Monitoring instruments

Before the monitoring period for the evaluation began in April 1994, it was agreed by PSI with each of the MGPs that monitoring information would be completed for first consultations, subsequent antenatal consultations with MGP midwives (these were called second and subsequent consultations) and the outcome of each pregnancy. The first consultation or booking form covered information such as age, marital status, ethnic group and housing status, the occupation of the woman and, where relevant, her partner. Information on the source of referral, the woman's GP, outcome and location of previous pregnancies, number of weeks gestation at booking and expected date of delivery was also collected. It was important to determine the choices women were offered, what they chose and the reasons why women were not offered choices about such aspects of care as lead professional and preferred place of birth. Where discussions about mode of delivery and labour preferences had taken place, the woman's preferences were recorded. Referrals to GPs and consultant obstetricians, any special points discussed and the length of each consultation were also recorded.

All antenatal consultation forms (first consultation and second and subsequent forms) requested information on the location of the consultation and the midwife seen in order to determine the extent to which women had received continuity of care and carer. Shorter forms were completed for each second and subsequent consultation with an MGP midwife, giving details of changes made by the woman in relation to lead professional, place of birth, mode of delivery and labour preferences. Details of referrals to GPs and consultant obstetricians were also recorded, as well as special points discussed and the length of the consultation.

Information was also recorded on the outcome of each pregnancy, confirming all maternities, miscarriages, terminations of pregnancy, and whether clients left the scheme or moved out of the area before delivery. Further information on all maternities was collected on the birthweight and sex of each live baby, the number of weeks gestation at delivery, location of delivery and full details of care received during labour, delivery and the postnatal period up to discharge from MGP care.

Activity levels of the MGPs during the monitoring period

First we present Table 3.1 which shows the number of women who were cared for by the MGPs in the monitoring period 1 April 1994 to 30 September 1995. During the monitoring period details of all antenatal consultations and pregnancy outcomes were recorded by the MGPs. The monitoring exercise was complicated by the fact that none of the MGPs started from scratch – each MGP brought a number of women with them into the evaluation who were at various stages in their pregnancies, having booked with the midwives from one to five months before the start of the evaluation. Monitoring information was also collected for this group of women (referred to as a 'reference group') to provide a complete picture of the activity and workload of individual midwives and the MGPs. All these women had delivered by the end of October 1994, after which time the midwives provided care solely to women who had booked with them within the period of the evaluation.

Table 3.1   Monitoring information completed by MGP midwives for all
women who received MGP care

numbers

	Pre-April 1994 women				Post-April 1994 women			
	Total	Lew	Ash	Dept	Total	Lew	Ash	Dept
First consultation booking forms	450	146	234	70	1,221	498	555	168
Second and subsequent consultation forms	2,086	690	964	432	6,763	3,098	2,765	900
Outcome forms	427	140	225	62	795	345	337	113
Total number of monitoring forms	(2,963)	(976)	(1,423)	(564)	(8,779)	(3,941)	(3,657)	(1,181)

Information on women who had received some of their care before April 1994

Information was collected for 146 women in Lewisham, 234 in Ashford and 70 in Deptford who had booked with midwives in the MGP before 1 April 1994, many of whom had already received a significant amount of antenatal care. The first consultation details, although collected at a relatively advanced point in pregnancy for many women, give a good indication of the background and characteristics of women who were also receiving MGP care for the first six to seven months of the evaluation. Outcome records were completed which provided information on the intrapartum and postnatal care provided by the MGPs. However, we will not be referring in detail to the care as such, other than to mention how and to what extent it formed part of the MGP's activity and workload. A profile of these service users with their main characteristics and outcome details is presented in Appendix C. It provides useful comparative information with the main group of women booked by the MGPs during the monitoring period.

Information on women who booked with the MGPs after April 1994

The focus of our analysis and discussion in this chapter and in Chapter 4 will concentrate on women who booked with the MGPs after April 1994, primarily because the MGP services were established to provide care for these women which makes them central to the overall evaluation. Women in this post-April 1994 group had, by and large, received only MGP care, but more importantly they had been offered choices and care options not offered to the other group of women, who had booked before April 1994. It is this feature that distinguishes this post-April 1994 group of women, and it is these differences that are drawn upon in interviews carried out with the women themselves which will be discussed more fully in Chapters 5 and 6.

Over the 18-month monitoring period from April 1994 to September 1995, booking information was collected for 1,221 women from the three MGPs – 498 women in Lewisham, 555 in Ashford and 168 in Deptford. 10 per cent of the women had received care elsewhere and then transferred to one of the MGPs for the remainder of their care in pregnancy but the majority of women booked with the MGP, usually in early pregnancy, and received a full episode of care from the point of booking until discharge from MGP care.

Number of bookings carried out by MGPs between 1 April 1994 and 30 September 1995

We looked at the monthly booking rate for the MGPs and each of the midwives between 1 April 1994 and 30 September 1995 in order to get a clear indication of the workload distribution both within and between the practices. These data are presented in Table 3.2, 3.3 and 3.4. The tables should be looked at together for comparative purposes because they reveal some important differences across the three areas.

The layout of the tables require a brief explanation for ease of understanding. The number of monthly bookings for each named midwife is presented in the columns of data on each table. The first total column shows the number and proportion of bookings for each midwife over the 18-month period from April 1994 to September 1995. We then show the totals for the three six-month periods which make up the whole, in order to give some indication of the trends over the monitoring period.

Lewisham MGP bookings

Table 3.2 clearly shows that the Lewisham MGP booked more women per annum than they had planned to deliver if they intended to keep to their target of 240 deliveries per annum. For instance, the total number of MGP bookings for the first twelve months of the evaluation from April 1994 to the end of March 1995 was 336 (28 per month). In fact the booking rate for the entire 18-month monitoring period was quite steady. The total number of bookings was 498 (28 per month).

The average number of bookings per midwife for the first 12 months of the monitoring period was 48 (4 bookings per month) but the number of actual bookings for individual midwives ranged from 42 to 55.

Table 3.2 Number of monthly bookings for named midwives in Lewisham MGP

numbers and percentages

Named midwife	Total April '94 – Sept '95	A	M	J	J	A	S	Sub total April – Sept '94	O	N	D	J	F	M	Sub total Oct '94 March '95	A	M	J	J	A	S	Sub total April – Sept '95
Midwife 1	78 16%	5	4	3	2	7	5	26 16%	5	2	7	5	4	6	29 17%	5	3	5	4	5	1	23 14%
Midwife 2	71 14%	3	2	3	6	7	2	23 14%	4	5	0	7	4	1	21 12%	5	5	4	3	6	4	27 17%
Midwife 3	77 15%	5	4	1	5	2	6	23 14%	5	5	5	4	5	4	28 16%	1	10	2	4	5	4	26 16%
Midwife 4	65 13%	1	6	2	4	2	7	22 14%	1	6	1	4	3	5	20 11%	3	4	4	4	3	5	23 14%
Midwife 5	66 13%	2	5	4	3	4	3	21 13%	5	9	2	4	1	4	25 14%	4	4	2	2	2	6	20 13%
Midwife 6	78 16%	2	4	7	2	6	2	23 14%	3	7	4	4	4	5	27 16%	5	4	4	4	5	6	28 17%
Midwife 7	63 13%	3	4	2	7	4	4	24 15%	2	3	3	8	4	4	24 14%	3	1	1	3	5	2	15 9%
Base: MGP bookings	(498)							(162)							(174)							(162)

Ashford MGP bookings

The major difference between Lewisham and Ashford was that the monthly booking rate in Ashford changed dramatically after the first 12 months of the evaluation to coincide with the introduction of the JACANES II group of midwives who took on the care of high-risk women from March 1995. Table 3.3 shows that the total number of MGP bookings for the 18-month monitoring period was 555 (31 per month). However, the number of MGP bookings for the first 12 months was 419 (35 per month) but for the final six months the mean monthly booking rate had fallen to 23 per month.

The difference in booking rates between Lewisham and Ashford is very clear. In the first 12 months of the evaluation the Ashford MGP (with 6 midwives) booked around 25 per cent more women than Lewisham (with 7 midwives). In contrast, a drop-off in bookings in Ashford in the final six months and a steady booking rate in Lewisham resulted in the Lewisham MGP booking nearly 20 per cent more women than Ashford for this six-month period (April–September 1995).

In calculating the average number of bookings per Ashford midwife for the monitoring period, the number of midwives has been taken as six because one midwife replaced another who went on maternity leave. The average number of bookings for the six midwives over the first 12 months was 70 and the monthly booking rate was just under 6 per midwife. In contrast, the average monthly booking rate in the final six months of the evaluation was just under 4 per midwife, similar to the Lewisham booking rate.

It is possible to see the big differences between the midwives' workload within the Ashford MGP by looking at the number of bookings for individual midwives which ranged from 65 to 114 for the 18-month monitoring period. A grade G midwife covering Practice A.C (a four-handed partnership and a single-handed GP practice), had the highest number of bookings, (114), accounting for over one fifth of all MGP bookings. However a grade F midwife booked 108 women from Practice A.E (two single-handed GP practices), accounting for almost the same proportion of all the MGP bookings. 29 per cent of all the women booking with the MGP came through Practice A.B (a six-handed partnership) in which two midwives were based: the grade G midwife booked 95 women and the grade F midwife booked 65 women.

These figures clearly demonstrate the difficulty in maintaining equity of workload if there are differences in the number of women coming through the GP practices themselves. The question of midwives' grading and support arrangements should be reviewed in the light of this fact.

Table 3.3 Number of monthly bookings for named midwives in Ashford MGP

numbers and percentages

Named midwife	Total April '94 – Sept '95	A	M	J	J	A	S	Sub total April – Sept '94	O	N	D	J	F	M	Sub total Oct '94 March '95	A	M	J	J	A	S	Sub total April – Sept '95
Midwife 1	78 14%	1	9	7	3	7	4	31 14%	7	4	4	6	2	2	25 13%	3	5	6	2	3	3	22 16%
Midwife 2	108 19%	9	6	3	15	6	10	49 22%	6	4	8	6	6	5	35 18%	2	3	4	5	4	6	24 18%
Midwife 3	95 17%	8	4	5	6	6	8	37 16%	7	7	7	6	4	5	36 18%	2	5	6	4	2	3	22 16%
Midwife 4	47 8%	7	3	6	10	9	3	38 17%	3	1	0	0	0	0	4 2%	0	0	0	0	0	5	5 3%
Midwife 5	114 21%	7	7	11	7	7	6	45 20%	7	8	2	9	9	8	43 22%	3	2	5	5	4	7	26 19%
Midwife 6	65 12%	3	3	1	4	10	5	26 12%	5	6	2	5	3	2	23 12%	0	2	3	5	4	2	16 12%
Midwife 7	48 9%	0	0	0	0	0	0	0	0	5	10	5	5	2	27 14%	3	4	5	5	1	3	21 16%
Base: MGP bookings	(555)							(226)							(193)							(136)

Deptford MGP bookings

Table 3.4 shows that the picture for Deptford was very different. The total number of bookings for the 18-month monitoring period was 168 and the mean number of monthly bookings was only just over 9 for the whole MGP, compared with 28 for Lewisham and 31 for Ashford. The difficulties experienced by the Deptford MGP in negotiating funding and ensuring an adequate quota of referrals were more acute in the first 12 months of the monitoring period.

The total number of Deptford MGP bookings for the first 12 months was 77 (6.4 MGP bookings per month). This differs markedly from the Ashford MGP, whose booking rate was around five and a half times greater, and the Lewisham MGP, whose booking rate was four and a half times greater. The Deptford MGP had in fact booked only 12 women in the first three months of the evaluation. When funding difficulties became acute the MGP stopped taking bookings in mid-August 1994, having booked only 41 women since the beginning of the monitoring period in April 1994. Bookings were not taken in September 1994 and 29 women were booked with the MGP in the five-month period between October 1994 and the end of February 1995.

However, following the negotiation of a new contract with the local Health Commissioning agencies, the MGP booked 91 women for the final six months of the evaluation from April to September 1995 (15 per month). Even after the number of bookings had increased the difference in the MGP booking rates for the three areas was still evident. For instance, the Lewisham MGP had a booking rate which was around 75 per cent higher than Deptford and the Ashford booking rate was 50 per cent higher, reinforcing the persistent workload and caseload differences.

Bookings, deliveries and workload

One of the criteria laid down by SETRHA was that the MGPs should deliver 200 women per annum. However, it is clear that the number of deliveries per annum does not properly reflect the workload of the MGPs. A true picture of the activity and workload of the MGPs cannot be obtained by taking account of deliveries alone, not only because of the differences in organising and providing care that existed between the MGPs but also because of the difference between the number of bookings and the number of deliveries.

Throughout our collection and analysis of data we have always distinguished between women who had booked with midwives in the MGPs before April 1994 and those who booked after that date. In proposing to deliver up to 200 women per annum it was clear that women who had already booked with midwives within the MGPs would inevitably be included in this figure. Therefore, the total number of deliveries for the duration of the monitoring period also includes women who had booked

Table 3.4 Number of monthly bookings for named midwives in Deptford MGP

numbers and percentages

Named midwife	Total April '94 – Sept '95	A	M	J	J	A	S	Sub total April – Sept '94	O	N	D	J	F	M	Sub total Oct '94 March '95	A	M	J	J	A	S	Sub total April – Sept '95
Midwife 1	37 22%	0	1	2	1	4	0	8 20%	0	3	3	0	3	5	14 39%	1	3	5	2	2	2	15 16%
Midwife 2	10 6%	2	0	1	3	2	0	8 20%	1	0	1	0	0	0	2 6%	LE	F	T	M	G	P	0 0%
Midwife 3	39 23%	0	1	2	2	1	0	6 14%	0	1	1	1	1	0	4 11%	10	3	7	3	1	5	29 32%
Midwife 4	33 20%	0	0	1	2	3	0	6 14%	0	2	1	2	0	0	5 14%	6	1	3	4	3	5	22 24%
Midwife 5	21 13%	0	0	0	0	0	0	0 0%	1	1	3	0	2	2	9 25%	2	3	1	1	0	2	12 13%
Midwife 7	7 4%	0	0	0	5	0	0	5 12%	1	0	0	1	0	0	2 6%	LE	F	T	M	G	P	0 0%
Midwife 8	8 5%	1	0	1	4	2	0	8 20%	0	0	0	0	0	0	0 0%	LE	F	T	M	G	P	0 0%
Midwife 9	13 8%	0	0	0	0	0	0	0 0%	0	0	0	0	0	0	0 0%	2	4	2	1	4	0	13 14%
Base: MGP bookings	(168)							(41)							(36)							(91)

with the midwives before April 1994 but delivered within the period of the evaluation. At the start of the monitoring period in April 1994 all the MGPs were providing care to women who had booked with the midwives at some point between October 1993 and March 1994 (see Appendix C). All these women had delivered by October or November 1994. The information collected on this group of women allows us to draw some conclusions about the activity and workload of the MGPs.

Looking at the Lewisham MGP first, Table 3.5 shows the total number of deliveries for women who booked before or after April 1994 and delivered at some stage in the first 12 months of the monitoring period. Outcome records were completed for 304 deliveries for this 12-month period, which was over 25 per cent more women than the MGP was set up to care for. 46 per cent of the deliveries related to women who had booked with midwives before April 1994 and the remainder were women who had booked with the MGP within the monitoring period. The total number of deliveries for the 18-month period was 454. It must be remembered that 20 of the 304 women delivered in other hospitals and therefore did not have a Lewisham MGP midwife in attendance (but could still receive antenatal and postnatal MGP care). The figures for all deliveries over the whole monitoring period indicate that the number of women who chose to deliver in another hospital was not predictable and in fact fell markedly in the last six months from 1 April 1995 to 30 September 1995. It is clear that a steady booking rate coupled with a drop in the proportion of women choosing to deliver elsewhere would have workload implications for the Lewisham MGP.

Table 3.5 shows that the Ashford MGP recorded 389 deliveries for the first 12 months of the monitoring period. 57 per cent of the women who delivered in the first 12 months had booked with one of the MGP midwives before April 1994 while the remainder booked within the monitoring period. The total number of deliveries for the 18-month period was 510. Not all these women were delivered by MGP midwives if they were under the care of a consultant obstetrician or if they had booked to deliver in another hospital. In contrast, the Deptford MGP was operating well below its expected capacity and recorded only 105 deliveries over the first 12 months of the monitoring period. 59 per cent of the women who had delivered in the first 12 months had booked with one of the MGP midwives before April 1994 while the remainder booked within the monitoring period. The total number of deliveries was 164 over the full 18-month monitoring period.

Table 3.5 Monthly deliveries for all MGPs during the monitoring period

numbers and percentages

	Total April '94 – Sept '95	A	M	J	J	A	S	Sub total April – Sept '94	O	N	D	J	F	M	Sub total Oct '94 – March '95	A	M	J	J	A	S	Sub total April – Sept '95
Lewisham																						
Pre-April 1994 MGP bookings	140	25	19	20	25	24	19	132	8	0	0	0	0	0	8	0	0	0	0	0	0	0
Post-April 1994 MGP bookings	314	0	0	1	1	3	5	10	19	31	19	30	29	26	154	54	20	28	31	26	21	150
Base: monitoring period deliveries	*(454)*							*(142)*							*(162)*							*(150)*
Ashford																						
Pre-April 1994 MGP bookings	223	28	40	45	35	24	26	198	18	7	0	0	0	0	25	0	0	0	0	0	0	0
Post-April 1994 MGP bookings	287	0	0	0	1	2	4	7	9	28	34	32	32	24	159	21	21	20	19	25	15	121
Base: monitoring period deliveries	*(510)*							*(205)*							*(184)*							*(121)*
Deptford																						
Pre-April 1994 MGP bookings	62	5	10	10	13	11	8	57	4	1	0	0	0	0	5	0	0	0	0	0	0	0
Post-April 1994 MGP bookings	102	0	0	0	1	1	2	4	4	4	11	6	9	5	39	4	17	12	7	10	9	59
Base: monitoring period deliveries	*(164)*							*(61)*							*(44)*							*(59)*

Characteristics of service users who booked with MGP midwives between 1 April 1994 and 30 September 1995

Age profile of users

Table 3.6 shows the age profile of women using the MGP services in the three areas. One of the most notable differences emerging from the table was the age profile of the women using the MGP service in Deptford compared with both Lewisham and Ashford. The average age of women booking with the Deptford MGP was 31.8 years compared with Lewisham (28.4 years) and Ashford (27.5 years). Around a quarter of women booking with the Lewisham MGP (23 per cent) and 29 per cent of women in Ashford were under 25 compared with only 13 per cent of women in Deptford. 14 per cent of women booking with the Deptford MGP were 25-29 year olds compared to just over one third (35 per cent) in Lewisham and Ashford.

A clear message from Table 3.6 is that the Deptford MGP attracted a much higher proportion of women over 30 than the other MGPs. Nearly three-quarters of the women in Deptford booking with the MGP were over 30 (74 per cent) compared with only one third in Ashford (36 per cent) and 42 per cent in Lewisham.

Table 3.6   Age of women booking with the MGPs

column percentages

	Lewisham	Ashford	Deptford
16-19	5	7	6
20-24	18	22	7
25-29	35	35	14
30-34	29	27	42
35-39	11	8	26
40 plus	2	1	6
n.a.	1	*	0
Mean age	*28.4*	*27.5*	*31.8*
Base: all MGP bookings	*(498)*	*(555)*	*(168)*

* equals less than 1 per cent

Marital status

Table 3.7 shows the differences in marital status across the projects. The big difference was in Ashford where over two-thirds (69 per cent) of women were married, compared with over a half (53 per cent) in

Lewisham and less than a half (49 per cent) in Deptford. A much higher proportion of women in Lewisham (22 per cent) and Deptford (21 per cent) were single, compared to only 8 per cent in Ashford. Just over a fifth of women in Lewisham and Ashford and over one quarter in Deptford were living as married. Only a small number of women in all areas were either divorced or separated.

Table 3.7   Marital status of women booking with the MGPs

column percentages

	Lewisham	Ashford	Deptford
Single	22	8	21
Married	53	69	49
Living as married	22	21	27
Widowed	*	0	0
Divorced	*	2	1
Separated	2	1	1
n.a.	0	0	1
Base: all MGP bookings	*(498)*	*(555)*	*(168)*

Social class and occupation

a)   *Women's occupation*

We collected data on occupation for both the women booking with the MGPs and their partners, although, as expected, information was not always supplied on partner's occupation.

Table 3.8 shows clearly that women in Deptford were much more likely to be in professional and managerial occupations (47 per cent) than women in Lewisham (23 per cent) and Ashford (19 per cent). Women in skilled non-manual occupations featured more in Lewisham (27 per cent) and Ashford (22 per cent) than in Deptford (8 per cent). Only a small proportion of women in all areas were in skilled manual occupations or semi-skilled and unskilled occupations.

Women in Ashford were twice as likely (37 per cent) to report being a housewife or mother than women in Deptford (18 per cent), while over a quarter of women (26 per cent) reported this in Lewisham. The proportion of women who were unemployed or students was noticeably higher in Deptford. 15 per cent of women in Deptford were unemployed compared with 9 per cent in Lewisham and 5 per cent in Ashford. However, it should be noted that the recording of occupations such as housewife and unemployed may be different within and between the three areas, depending both on the interpretation of midwives and the women themselves, so that one woman might say she was a housewife but could equally claim to be unemployed or vice versa.

Table 3.8   Social class/occupation of women booking with MGPs and their partners

column percentages

	Women			Partners		
	Lew	Ash	Dept	Lew	Ash	Dept
Professional I	1	2	4	5	6	10
Intermediate II	22	17	43	19	22	39
Skilled non-manual III N	27	22	8	12	9	8
Skilled manual III M	5	4	2	33	25	11
Semi-skilled IV	5	8	2	6	12	4
Unskilled V	1	2	1	4	6	2
Student	3	2	6	3	2	2
Armed Forces	0	0	0	0	*	0
Keeping house/Mother	26	37	18	*	*	0
Unemployed	9	5	15	9	12	13
Retired	0	0	0	*	0	0
n.a.	*	2	0	7	5	11
Base: all MGP bookings	*(498)*	*(555)*	*(168)*	*(498)*	*(555)*	*(168)*

b) *Partner's occupation*

Table 3.8 underlines the differences between Deptford and elsewhere. Nearly half of the partners in Deptford (49 per cent) were in professional and managerial occupations, compared with 28 per cent of partners in Ashford and 24 per cent in Lewisham. 43 per cent of partners in Ashford and Lewisham were in manual occupations compared with 17 per cent of partners in Deptford. In fact, the most commonly reported occupational category for partners in both Lewisham (33 per cent) and Ashford (25 per cent) were the skilled manual occupations, while in Deptford more partners reported being in managerial occupations (39 per cent) than any other occupation.

Roughly the same proportion of partners in Deptford and Ashford were reported to be unemployed (13 and 12 per cent) which was slightly higher than in Lewisham (9 per cent). The relatively high number of 'not applicable' responses could be attributed to the fact that some women did not see themselves as having partners, although it is also clearly due to a reluctance by midwives to ask about partners if they felt a pregnancy was unintended.

Ethnic group

Information on ethnic group was collected for women who booked with the MGPs. While two of the projects exhibited some ethnic diversity, Table 3.9 clearly indicates that an overwhelming majority of women booked by all MGPs were of white ethnic origin. The Ashford MGP booked the highest proportion of white women (96 per cent) compared with Lewisham (77 per cent) and Deptford (73 per cent).

23 per cent of the women who booked with the Lewisham MGP were from a number of different ethnic minority groups but 18 per cent of all bookings were from Black minority groups alone.

The Ashford MGP exhibited less ethnic diversity than either of the London-based MGPs. 1 per cent of women booking with the MGP were described as Black African, 1 per cent were Middle Eastern and a further 1 per cent were Indian.

26 per cent of the women who booked with the Deptford MGP were from non-white ethnic minority groups and 15 per cent of women were from Black minority groups alone. 2 per cent were Indian, 1 per cent Bangladeshi and 1 per cent Chinese. The proportion of Vietnamese women booking with the Deptford MGP (4 per cent) was not surprising given the large Vietnamese community living in Deptford.

Table 3.9 Ethnic group of women booking with the MGPs

column percentages

	Lewisham	Ashford	Deptford
White	77	96	73
Black Caribbean	11	*	10
Black African	7	1	4
Black British	*	*	1
Indian	1	1	2
Pakistani	*	*	0
Bangladeshi	*	0	1
Chinese	*	0	1
Vietnamese	0	*	4
Mixed race	3	*	2
Middle Eastern	0	1	1
Other	1	*	1
Base: all MGP bookings	*(498)*	*(555)*	*(168)*

Housing status

We included a question on housing status on the first consultation form which was used at a later stage to identify any links between women's preferences for place of birth and their own housing circumstances. For instance, a home birth may not have been as realistic an option for women who lived in temporary accommodation or with relatives, compared with other women who owned the accommodation in which they lived.

Table 3.10 shows the housing status of all the women who booked with the MGPs. While there were some differences, especially in relation to the proportion of ownership in the three areas, there was also much similarity in tenancy status and other living circumstances of the women in general. The highest proportion of owner occupation was in Ashford and Deptford where over half the women (55 per cent) were reported as owner-occupiers, compared with less than half the women in Lewisham.

Roughly the same proportion of women in the three areas were private and council tenants, although the proportion of council tenancy in Lewisham was higher than elsewhere. 9 per cent of women in Lewisham were living with relatives compared with 6 per cent in Ashford and 3 per cent in Deptford. A small proportion of women in all areas were described as living with a friend or partner, living in temporary accommodation or living in a hotel/hostel. In some instances, especially in Deptford, it was reported by midwives that living arrangements were short-term or uncertain which might leave a number of women homeless. However, to ensure consistency in analysis, housing status was determined on the basis of actual accommodation at booking, however uncertain or temporary it was thought to be.

Table 3.10 Housing status of women booking with the MGPs

column percentages

	Lewisham	Ashford	Deptford
Owner-occupier	49	55	55
Private tenant	11	12	11
Council tenant	25	21	20
Hotel or hostel	1	1	2
Living with relatives	9	6	3
Housing Association	2	1	4
Temporary address	1	1	1
Other living arrangements	1	1	1
n.a.	*	2	3
Base: all MGP bookings	(498)	(555)	(168)

Number and outcome of previous pregnancies

Table 3.11 shows that 30 per cent of women in Lewisham and 29 per cent in Ashford reported being pregnant for the first time compared with 20 per cent in Deptford. One third of women in each of the three areas had had one previous pregnancy and nearly one fifth of women in all areas had had two previous pregnancies. 25 per cent of women in Deptford and around one fifth in Ashford and Lewisham had had three or more previous pregnancies.

Table 3.11 Number of previous pregnancies for women booking with the MGPs

column percentages

	Lewisham	Ashford	Deptford
Number of previous pregnancies			
None	30	29	20
1	33	33	33
2	16	20	21
3 plus	20	17	25
n.a.	0	0	1
Base: GP bookings	*(468)*	*(555)*	*(168)*

We were interested in the number of previous maternities – live and still-births – as well as previous miscarriages, terminations of pregnancy and ectopic pregnancies. Tables 3.12 and 3.13 show that there were marked differences in outcomes for women in the three areas with a higher proportion of miscarriages, terminations of pregnancy (TOPs), ectopic pregnancies and stillbirths for women in Deptford. It should be noted that the numbers in Deptford overall were small.

Previous maternities

Previous live births over 37 weeks – Table 3.12 shows that over one third of women in each area had had one previous live birth over 37 weeks. Nearly one sixth of women in each area had had two previous live births, and less than 10 per cent had had three or more live births.

Previous live births under 37 weeks – around 5 per cent of women in each area had had one pre-term live birth while another 1 per cent in each area had had two pre-term live births.

Stillbirths – 2 per cent of women in Deptford had had one previous stillbirth, 1 per cent in Lewisham and less than 1 per cent in Ashford. One woman in Lewisham had had two previous stillbirths.

Table 3.12 Number of previous maternities for women booking with the MGPs

column percentages

	Live births over 37 weeks			Live births under 37 weeks			Stillbirths		
	Lew	Ash	Dept	Lew	Ash	Dept	Lew	Ash	Dept
None	44	42	40	94	95	96	99	99	98
One	34	35	36	5	4	4	1	*	2
Two	13	15	16	1	1	1	*	0	0
Three or more	8	7	7	0	*	0	0	0	0
Base: all MGP bookings	(498)	(555)	(168)	(498)	(555)	(168)	(498)	(555)	(168)

Overall, nearly the same proportion of women in the three areas were parous (62 per cent in Deptford, 61 per cent in Ashford and 59 per cent in Lewisham). It is interesting to note the difference between the proportion of women who had had one or more previous *live or stillbirths* and the proportion who had had one or more previous *pregnancies* (79 per cent in Deptford, 70 per cent in Ashford and 69 per cent in Lewisham). The marked difference in the figures for Deptford – 79 per cent with a previous pregnancy and 62 per cent with a previous live or stillbirth – can be attributed to the higher incidence of miscarriages and terminations of pregnancy recorded among the Deptford women.

Previous neonatal deaths – a slightly higher proportion of women in Deptford (3 per cent) had had a baby who died between birth and 27 days compared with Lewisham and Ashford (1 per cent or less).

Other previous pregnancies

Miscarriages – Table 3.13 shows that nearly one third of women in Deptford reported previous miscarriages compared with around one fifth of women in Ashford and Lewisham. 23 per cent of women in Deptford had had one previous miscarriage compared with 18 per cent in Lewisham and 16 per cent in Ashford. 9 per cent of women in Deptford had had two or more previous miscarriages compared with 3 per cent in Lewisham and 4 per cent in Ashford.

Terminations of pregnancy – the most marked difference between women in Deptford and elsewhere was that 27 per cent reported ever having had a termination of pregnancy (TOP) compared with 15 per cent in Lewisham and 11 per cent in Ashford. Women in Deptford were twice as likely to have had one TOP (22 per cent) than women in Ashford (10 per cent) and Lewisham (12 per cent). 5 per cent of women in Deptford had had two or more TOPs compared with only 1 per cent in Ashford and 3 per cent in Lewisham.

Ectopic pregnancy – a slightly higher proportion of women in Deptford (2 per cent) had had a previous ectopic pregnancy than in Lewisham (less than 1 per cent) and Ashford (1 per cent).

Table 3.13 Number of previous miscarriages, terminations of pregnancy and ectopic pregnancies for women booking with the MGPs

column percentages

| | Outcome of previous pregnancies | | | | | | | | |
| | Miscarriages | | | TOPs | | | Ectopics | | |
	Lew	Ash	Dept	Lew	Ash	Dept	Lew	Ash	Dept
None	79	80	69	85	89	73	99	99	98
One	18	16	23	12	10	22	*	1	2
Two	2	3	7	2	1	3	0	0	0
Three or more	1	1	2	1	0	2	0	0	0
Base: all MGP bookings	*(498)*	*(555)*	*(168)*	*(498)*	*(555)*	*(168)*	*(498)*	*(555)*	*(168)*

General practitioners and GP practices taking part in the evaluation

In order to see if some GPs were more actively involved in providing maternity care than others we asked midwives to record the name of the woman's GP on each first consultation form. We found that within the GP practices a few GPs provided a greater proportion of maternity care. However, the uneven distribution of women to GPs was more notable in Lewisham than elsewhere.

Lewisham GP practices

17 GPs were listed as the named GP for women booking with the Lewisham MGP, which is somewhat surprising because locum and trainee GPs should not have been the named GP for any of the women. However, this may have been the result of a lack of understanding on the part of the midwives themselves rather than a reflection of actual practice. Twelve GPs (one of whom left during the monitoring period) were based in the three GP practices taking part in the evaluation – 6 in Practice L.A, 3 in Practice L.B and 3 in Practice L.C.

Looking at the number of women receiving maternity care from each GP practice, nearly half of all the women booking with the MGP were from Practice L.A (48 per cent), compared to 28 per cent of the women from Practice L.B and 22 per cent from Practice L.C. This may explain why some of the midwives in Practice L.C had to book women from Practice L.A to ensure more equity in midwifery caseload and workload.

Within the GP practices themselves we found that maternity care was the responsibility of only a few GPs:

- In Practice L.A, one GP alone was the named GP for over half of the maternity caseload for the practice and nearly one quarter of all the women booking with the MGP. Another two GPs were named GPs for 31 per cent and 14 per cent of the women in the practice, while the remaining three GPs were named GP for fewer than five women each.

- In Practice L.B, one GP was named GP for nearly two-thirds of the women registered with the practice, another GP had over one third of the women and a part-time GP was named GP for two women.

- In Practice L.C, one GP was named GP for 80 per cent of the women within the practice and nearly one quarter of the women booking with the MGP overall. Another GP had 20 per cent of the women and the third member of the practice was named GP for nine women.

Ashford GP practices

In Ashford 28 GPs were recorded as a named GP for women who had booked with the MGP, 7 of whom were not permanent members of the five GP practices taking part in the evaluation and 2 of whom left during the monitoring period.

This left 19 GPs in the five GP 'host practices'. 4 GPs were based at Practice A.A; 6 at Practice A.B; 4 at Practice A.C; 2 at Practice A.D; and 2 single-handed GPs in Practice A.E. One other single-handed GP practice was covered by the midwife based at Practice A.C.

Although, as expected, some of the bigger practices had more women from the MGP registered with them, this was less marked than in Lewisham. 28 per cent of the women who had booked with the MGP were registered with the A.B Practice, 20 per cent with the single-handed GPs (Practice A.E), 18 per cent with Practice A.C, 16 per cent with Practice A.D, 12 per cent with Practice A.A and 3 per cent with the single-handed practice covered by A.C.

Within the GP practices some GPs were again more actively involved in providing maternity care than others:

- In Practice A.A, two GPs were named GP for 90 per cent of the women and the part-time GPs for the remainder.

- In Practice A.B, four GPs were the named GP for between one fifth and a quarter of women each while the other two were named GP for very few women.

- In Practice A.C, the female GP was named GP for 43 per cent of the women, another two GPs were named GP for between one fifth and a quarter of women and the fourth GP was named GP for the remainder.

- In Practice A.D, one GP was named GP for 87 per cent of the women and the other was named GP for the remainder.

- In Practice A.E, one of the two single-handed GPs was named GP for over half the women (54 per cent).

Deptford GP practices

The major difference between the Deptford MGP and elsewhere was that the midwives were not based at GP practices and were therefore responsible for engaging referrals themselves. While the MGP was independent of GPs in its set-up and practice, it was still expected that GPs would refer women to the service. There was a wider distribution of GPs noted in Deptford than in the other pilot areas and over 50 GPs were recorded as the named GP for women booking with the MGP. Only one GP was recorded as GP to more than 10 women, indicating a wider spread of women receiving MGP care in Deptford than elsewhere.

Table 3.14 Source of referral of women to the MGPs

column percentages

	Lewisham	Ashford	Deptford
GP	96	84	20
Self referral	2	14	62
Friends/relatives	0	0	13
Other community MW	1	1	4
Practice nurse	1	1	0
Health visitor	*	0	0
n.a.	0	*	1
Base: all MGP bookings	*(498)*	*(555)*	*(168)*

Details of current pregnancy

Access to the service – source of referral

Table 3.14 demonstrates clearly the differences in source of referral to the MGPs. In Lewisham almost all the women were referred to the MGP through their GP. It is interesting that in Ashford as many as 14 per cent of women self-referred to the MGP, mainly because they already knew some of the midwives from previous pregnancies. However, the big difference in source of referral was between Deptford and the other areas in that only 20 per cent of the Deptford women came through their GP and three-quarters self-referred or came through friends and relatives.

At what stage did women book their care with the MGPs?

We asked the midwives to record the number of weeks gestation for each woman at their first consultation or booking visit. It should be noted that booking refers to the first or initial booking consultation in pregnancy wherever it took place. As many as 42 per cent of the women who booked with the Deptford MGP after April 1994 had already booked elsewhere during their current pregnancy before transferring to MGP care.

Table 3.15 shows a remarkable difference between the booking pattern in Ashford and the other two MGPs, in that as many as two-thirds of all the women in Ashford had first booked their care at or before 10 weeks gestation compared to around a quarter of women booking in Lewisham and one fifth in Deptford. We also looked at the booking pattern both for women who had had previous pregnancies and those with no previous pregnancies which reinforced the differences already noted.

Table 3.15 Number of weeks gestation at first booking in pregnancy

column percentages

	Lewisham	Ashford	Deptford
Weeks gestation			
1-6	1	7	*
7-8	6	32	8
9-10	16	27	11
11-12	22	18	24
13-16	39	12	36
17-20	10	2	10
21-25	4	1	4
26+	2	1	4
n.a.	0	*	3
Base: all women receiving MGP care	(498)	(555)	(168)

In Ashford women who were pregnant for the first time did not necessarily book earlier than women who had had one or more previous pregnancies, which suggests that early booking was more likely to have resulted from the organisation of the first consultation or booking visits by the MGP itself.

In contrast, 60 per cent of women in Deptford who had had no previous pregnancies had originally booked their care at or before 12 weeks, compared with only around a third of women who had one previous pregnancy, 42 per cent who had two previous pregnancies and nearly half the women who had three or more previous pregnancies.

In Lewisham the proportion of women with no previous pregnancies who booked at or before 12 weeks was only a little higher than among women who had had previous pregnancies.

These differences in booking patterns are important because of the implications that booking arrangements could have for midwives' workload and women's expectations and perception of the care they received (see Chapters 5 and 6). In addition, the incidence of miscarriage in the three areas may in part be explained by the variations in booking patterns.

How many women had already received maternity care elsewhere in their current pregnancy?

42 per cent of the women who booked with the Deptford MGP during the monitoring period had received maternity care elsewhere during their current pregnancy. Women in Ashford and Lewisham were much more likely to have received all their care from the MGP, as only 4 per cent transferred to MGP care from elsewhere in Ashford and 7 per cent in Lewisham. This reinforces the point that the Deptford MGP attracted a different group of women, some of whom were not satisfied with the care they had received before their transfer to MGP care.

It was important to establish at what stage in pregnancy this happened and whether there were notable differences across the three areas. All the women who transferred to the MGPs did so after at least 10 weeks gestation. Around two-thirds of the women who transferred in Lewisham and Ashford did so at or before 30 weeks gestation, but, as noted above, transfers accounted for only very small proportions of the total women cared for by these two MGPs. We have seen that 42 per cent of all the women in Deptford had already received care elsewhere, but over 20 per cent of all women cared for by the Deptford midwives transferred to MGP care *after 31 weeks* and over 10 per cent of all women transferred *after 36 weeks.*

This has important implications for the workload of the three MGPs, as well as potential resource implications of double-counting of midwifery or maternity services. The amount of antenatal care involved in looking after women for the last 4 weeks or 9 weeks of their pregnancies is clearly much less than is involved in a full episode of midwifery care.

Choices in pregnancy

i) Lead professional

One of the objectives set out in *Changing Childbirth* was that women should be fully involved in making decisions about their care and should have a choice about who would look after them during their pregnancy. It also stated that 'a woman with an uncomplicated pregnancy, should if she wishes, be able to book with a midwife as the lead professional for the entire episode of care including delivery in a general hospital'. We asked the midwives to record whether women were offered a choice of lead professional and if not to give the reasons why.

Women in Lewisham were more likely to have been offered a choice (98 per cent) than women in Ashford (90 per cent) and Deptford (79 per cent). Table 3.16 shows that midwife-led care was overwhelmingly favoured by women in all areas. 98 per cent of the women who were offered a choice in Deptford opted for midwife-led care compared with 91 per cent in Lewisham and 71 per cent in Ashford. Consultant-led care was chosen by a fifth of women in Ashford and only a handful of women in Lewisham and Deptford. In contrast, GP-led and shared care arrangements were chosen by very few women in Ashford and Lewisham and by none of the women in Deptford. However, two of the women we interviewed in Deptford said that they had opted for a shared care arrangement between their midwife and GP which was not recorded on the first consultation forms.

Table 3.16 Choice of lead professional for women offered options at booking with the MGPs

column percentages

Options	Lewisham	Ashford	Deptford
MGP midwife	91	71	98
Consultant obstetrician	1	20	1
GP	1	*	0
Shared: CO/MW	1	2	0
Shared: GP/MW	2	2	0
Shared: GP/hospital	0	0	0
Shared: GP/MW/hospital	*	*	0
Undecided	0	4	0
No preference expressed	3	1	1
Base: all women offered choice of lead professional at booking	*(488)*	*(498)*	*(131)*

In Ashford there were clear protocols for assigning women to MGP care and consultant care which, if adhered to, would have resulted in high risk women not being offered the same choices about who would care for them during their pregnancy. However, the figures clearly show that 90 per cent of all the women who booked with the Ashford MGP were offered a choice of lead professional, and 71 per cent chose midwife-led care. This makes it difficult to explain the differences between cases where women were offered a choice (even though they may have been assessed as high risk) and chose a consultant obstetrician as lead professional, and those who were not given a choice and assigned a consultant obstetrician as lead professional because of their obstetric or medical requirements.

The issue of choice and the presentation of care options must be set against the fact that the MGPs were expected to deliver at least 200 women per annum which meant that it was taken as given that most of the women would receive midwife-led care anyway. Because of this pre-condition, care options might not have been presented on a level playing field thereby placing obvious constraints on choice from the outset. In addition, GP-led care and some forms of shared care arrangements could have been placed at a disadvantage because the force of organisation and expectation was that other options would prevail.

Why were women not offered a choice of lead professional?

In Deptford nearly all the women who were not given a choice were reported to have already decided who they wanted as lead professional which was not as prevalent in Ashford or Lewisham. The most common reason cited in Ashford and Lewisham for not giving women a choice was because of their previous obstetric or medical history.

ii) Place of birth

The objective set by *Changing Childbirth* on place of birth was that 'women should receive clear, unbiased advice and be able to choose where they would like their baby to be born. The right to make that choice should be respected and every practical effort made to achieve the outcome that the woman believes is best for her baby and herself.'

Midwives were asked to record on the first consultation form if women were offered a choice of place of birth, the option chosen by the woman and reasons for not offering a choice if relevant. 96 per cent of women in Lewisham were offered a choice of place of birth, 94 per cent in Ashford and 91 per cent in Deptford.

A key message which emerged here was the value that women placed on being able to choose where they wanted their baby to be born. Table 3.17 shows that all the women expressed a preference at booking or said that they would like to make a decision about place of birth at a later stage, indicating that being offered options and having the opportunity to choose where they wanted to deliver their baby was clearly important to them. However, it was interesting to see how many women did not feel they could make a decision on place of birth at the first consultation. As many as one fifth of women in Deptford did not decide compared with 8 per cent in Ashford and 4 per cent in Lewisham.

Table 3.17 shows the particular options chosen by women in the three areas. One of the major differences between Deptford and the other areas was the proportion of women who opted for a home birth. Over half of the women who were offered a choice in Deptford (52 per cent) chose a home birth, compared with only 12 per cent in Lewisham and 5 per cent in Ashford, indicating yet again that the Deptford MGP attracted women with different preferences from those in Lewisham and Ashford.

Table 3.17 **Preferred place of birth for women who were offered a choice at booking with the MGPs**

column percentages

	Lewisham	Ashford	Deptford
Home birth	12	5	52
Hospital – not DOMINO	34	16	5
Hospital – DOMINO	50	70	22
GP Unit	0	1	0
Undecided	4	8	21
No preference	0	0	0
Base: women offered choice of place of birth at booking	*(478)*	*(522)*	*(153)*

A similar proportion of women in Lewisham (84 per cent) and Ashford (86 per cent) chose to have their baby in hospital compared with just over a quarter of women in Deptford (27 per cent). Table 3.17 demonstrates that a DOMINO delivery was favoured by women in all areas who chose a hospital birth, but this was especially evident in Ashford. 70 per cent of the women offered a choice in Ashford chose a DOMINO delivery, compared with half of the women in Lewisham and just over one fifth in Deptford which supports and reinforces the views of women expressed in *Changing Childbirth* about their preference for DOMINO deliveries.

Why were women not given a choice of place of birth?

In Lewisham the most common reason cited for not offering women a choice of place of birth was because of their obstetric or medical history or because they were reported to have already decided what they wanted. In Ashford women were much more likely not to have been offered a choice because of an obstetric or medical history or because they were already booked at another hospital. In Deptford two-thirds of the women not offered a choice were reported to have already decided, and their preferred option was almost always a home birth, a quarter had a previous obstetric history of note and the remainder were already booked to deliver at a local hospital.

Housing status and chosen place of birth

It is possible that women's housing circumstances could have an influence on their choice of place of birth in that a home birth might not be seen as a realistic option for some women living in temporary accommodation or those living with relatives. Looking at housing status and preferred place of birth together we found that a higher proportion of women in all areas who expressed a preference for a home birth were owner-occupiers. Interviews with the women discussed in Chapters 5 and 6 reinforce the view that some women's housing and living circumstances dictated the choices they could make about where they would give birth.

In Lewisham 68 per cent of the women who opted for a home birth were owner-occupiers and 19 per cent were council tenants. Only 1 of the 43 women who were living with relatives and none of the women in temporary accommodation opted for a home birth.

Of the 24 women in Ashford who expressed a preference for a home birth, 14 were owner-occupiers, 6 were private tenants and 4 were council tenants. None of the 32 women who were living with relatives or in temporary accommodation opted for a home birth.

In Deptford, as in Lewisham, a high proportion of the women who opted for a home birth were owner-occupiers (60 per cent), 20 per cent were council tenants and the remainder were mostly private tenants or lived in housing association accommodation.

iii) Mode of delivery and labour preferences

In the discussion on care in labour, *Changing Childbirth* set out the objective that 'women should have the opportunity to discuss their plans for labour and birth. Their decisions should be recorded in their birth plans and incorporated into their case notes. Every reasonable effort should be made to accommodate the wishes of the woman and her partner, and to inform them of the services that are available to them.' We asked midwives to record if any initial discussion on mode of delivery had taken place at the first consultation and also to record the woman's preference regarding labour and mode of delivery.

Around three-quarters of women in Lewisham (79 per cent) and Deptford (73 per cent) and two-thirds in Ashford (64 per cent) discussed mode of delivery with their midwife at the first consultation. The majority of women who had discussed mode of delivery expressed a preference for a normal vaginal delivery which was as natural as possible (94 per cent in Deptford, 91 per cent in Lewisham and 89 per cent in Ashford). A handful of women discussed the possibility of having a caesarean section. The most common reason cited by midwives for not discussing mode of delivery was that it was felt to be too early, or that it was not necessary if the woman had had previous normal deliveries.

Women in Deptford were nearly twice as likely to express labour preferences (65 per cent) as women in Ashford (36 per cent). In Deptford women placed more emphasis on having a normal, natural labour with minimal intervention than women elsewhere, and also requested the opportunity to labour at home for as long as possible and to have an assessment by their midwife at home in early labour. It is interesting that hardly any of the women in Deptford expressed a preference for a pain-free labour with good pain control, and some women requested no or minimal analgesia. This would fit with the preference for minimal intervention and home births as a choice amongst this group of women, many of whom wished to have family and relatives around them.

Over half of the women in Lewisham (57 per cent) expressed labour preferences at their first consultation placing most emphasis on having a normal and natural labour with minimal intervention but this was less marked than in Deptford. A short pain-free labour was another preference expressed by women and specific pain relief options were often discussed.

In Ashford women placed most emphasis on being free to move around in labour and to alternate position or adopt preferred positions. While women did not specify a pain-free labour as such they did discuss pain relief in labour, being able to labour in water and preferred options for pain relief.

Did women change their preferences during pregnancy?

i) Lead professional

A tiny proportion of women in all areas (3 per cent in Lewisham, 6 per cent in Ashford and 5 per cent in Deptford) changed their lead professional at some point during pregnancy. In over half the cases in Lewisham the new lead professional was a consultant obstetrician and in the remainder of cases the new lead was an MGP midwife. In Deptford and Ashford most of the women changed lead professional to another MGP midwife, but in Ashford this was mainly attributed to one midwife going on maternity leave. A few women who developed complications during pregnancy changed lead professional to a consultant obstetrician.

ii) Place of birth

Less than 8 per cent of women in Lewisham and 5 per cent in Ashford changed their minds about their preferred place of birth or expressed a preference after a period of indecision. Most of the women concerned in Deptford had not made a decision about place of birth at their first consultation. Of those who changed or made up their minds, around half the women in Lewisham and Ashford and over a third of women in Deptford expressed a preference for a home birth, while the rest opted for a hospital birth. Second and subsequent monitoring forms often referred to discussions about changing place of birth and the value of keeping options open.

Access to information at the first consultation with the MGP

Throughout *Changing Childbirth* emphasis is placed over and over again on the value of communicating options to women, giving unbiased information which can inform their decisions and taking all the necessary steps to ensure that women feel fully supported and informed throughout their pregnancy. It was important to determine whether women were offered information on specific areas such as screening tests, pregnancy and childbirth. We asked midwives to record if women were offered information on these areas at their first consultation.

Telephone number of the named midwife: in all instances this information was given to women booking with the MGPs.

Oral and written information about antenatal screening: women were more likely to receive information about antenatal screening from discussions with the midwife rather than through written information in leaflets or books. A high proportion of women in all areas (98 per cent in Ashford, 95 per cent in Lewisham and 70 per cent in Deptford) discussed antenatal screening with their midwife. However, only 8 per cent of women in Deptford were offered additional written information, compared with 92 per cent of women in Lewisham and 84 per cent in Ashford. In Lewisham and Ashford leaflets on screening tests were specially drawn up to give to women booking with the MGPs.

Oral and written information about pregnancy and birth: 98 per cent of women in Lewisham, 88 per cent in Ashford and 93 per cent in Deptford discussed pregnancy and birth with their midwife. Again, the picture was very different in relation to written information in Deptford where only 4 per cent of women were offered written information, compared with 95 per cent of women in Lewisham and 92 per cent in Ashford.

What is surprising about the figures in Deptford is that the MGP had stressed the value of their information and library facilities, but their own forms clearly show that less than 10 per cent of the women booking with the MGP were offered written information on antenatal screening and less than 5 per cent of all women were offered information on pregnancy and birth at the first consultation with the MGP. In view of the fact that 42 per cent of all the women had received care elsewhere before transferring to the Deptford MGP, it is possible that some women had already received information about pregnancy and birth, and other information on screening tests may have been irrelevant if women transferred after a certain period in pregnancy. Nonetheless, the message which emerges from the figures is that the vast majority of women were not offered such information. 94 per cent of women who were pregnant for the first time did not receive any written information and this may be a cause for concern, particularly since they were more likely to have booked with the MGP within the first 12 weeks of pregnancy.

Location of consultations and time spent

a) First consultations or booking visits

We asked midwives to record the time spent with women at each first consultation. A major difference between Deptford and the other MGPs was that the Deptford midwives spent twice as long with women than midwives in Ashford and around 50 per cent more time on first consultations than midwives in Lewisham. The average length of first consultations in Deptford was 114 minutes, 78.1 minutes in Lewisham and 55.7 minutes in Ashford. Table 3.18 shows that 95 per cent of first consultations lasted over one hour in Deptford, compared to 72 per cent in Lewisham and only 19 per cent in Ashford.

Table 3.18 **Length of first consultation with women booking with the MGPs**

column percentages

	Lewisham	Ashford	Deptford
Length of consultation in minutes			
1-15	*	0	0
16-30	2	7	0
31-45	7	25	1
46-60	19	49	4
1 hour plus	72	19	95
n.a.	0	*	0
Mean number of minutes	*78.1*	*55.7*	*114.2*
Base: all first consultations with the MGPs	*(498)*	*(555)*	*(168)*

The next important difference was that first consultations were attended by one midwife only in Lewisham and Ashford but 22 per cent of all first consultations in Deptford were carried out by two midwives. This practice can be attributed to the fact that in Deptford a primary and secondary midwife booked and cared for each woman throughout pregnancy and for the birth of her baby. The relatively low booking rate in Deptford undoubtedly enabled two midwives to carry out first consultations and to spend this length of time with women. However, it is clear that if the MGP had booked the number of women set out in their proposal, this input of time and midwifery staff would have been unsustainable.

Table 3.19 shows the location of first consultations in each area. The shorter length of first consultations in Ashford could be attributed to the fact that 81 per cent of them took place at GP practices, while only 17 per cent of consultations occurred at home and 1 per cent at hospital.

This was completely different in Lewisham where 81 per cent of first consultations took place at the client's or a friend's home, only 12 per cent occurred at GP practices and 4 per cent at hospital.

In Deptford 92 per cent of booking consultations took place at the client's home, relative's or boyfriend's/ partner's home and 5 per cent took place at the Albany Centre (MGP office). 1 per cent took place at GP practices and 1 per cent at hospital.

Table 3.19 Location of first consultation with women booking with the MGPs

column percentages

	Lewisham	Ashford	Deptford
Client's home	81	17	88
GP surgery	12	81	*
Hospital	4	1	2
Albany Centre	0	0	5
Relative's/Partner's/ Friend's home	1	*	4
Other	*	0	1
n.a.	2	1	1
Base: all first consultations with the MGPs	*(498)*	*(555)*	*(168)*

b) Second and subsequent consultations

Midwives were asked to record the time spent on all second and subsequent consultations to determine the overall time spent with women on this aspect of antenatal care. As with first consultations, the major difference was that the average time spent by the Deptford midwives (68.8 minutes) was around twice as long as midwives in Lewisham (34.3 minutes) and two and one third times longer than by midwives in Ashford (28.8 minutes).

Table 3.20 shows the average length of second and subsequent consultations in each area. 78 per cent of second and subsequent consultations in Ashford lasted 30 minutes or less compared with 59 per cent of consultations in Lewisham and only 11 per cent in Deptford. Nearly half of all consultations in Deptford took between 31 and 60 minutes compared with over a third in Lewisham and less than a fifth in Ashford. 39 per cent of consultations in Deptford took over one hour compared with only 5 per cent in Lewisham and 3 per cent in Ashford.

Table 3.20 Length of second and subsequent consultations with women

column percentages

	Lewisham	Ashford	Deptford
Length of consultations in minutes			
1–15	4	17	1
16–30	55	61	10
31–45	26	13	18
46–60	9	6	31
1 hour plus	5	3	39
n.a.	*	*	*
Mean number of minutes	34.3	28.8	68.8
Base: all second and subsequent consultations	*(3,098)*	*(2,765)*	*(900)*

In addition, the Lewisham MGP carried out nearly three and a half times as many second and subsequent consultations (3,098 consultations) and the Ashford MGP carried out three times as many consultations (2,765 consultations) as the Deptford MGP (900 consultations). Only one midwife attended second and subsequent consultations in Lewisham and Ashford, but 7 per cent of all second and subsequent consultations in Deptford were attended by two midwives.

It is clear that the difference in time spent on consultations by the MGPs occurred because the Deptford MGP never operated at full capacity and therefore reflects the different demands on their service. It could be argued that any increase in caseload numbers by the Deptford MGP would have to be accompanied by a corresponding decrease in the time spent with women at consultations.

Accessible care: where did consultations take place?

The second principle underpinning woman centred care set out in *Changing Childbirth* relates to accessible care. It states that 'maternity care must be readily and easily accessible to all women. It should be sensitive to the needs of the local population and based primarily in the local community'. The MGPs were set up as community midwifery services and we were interested to determine where second and subsequent consultations had taken place in the three areas. Midwives were asked to record the location of each second and subsequent consultation on the monitoring forms. We have already seen from Table 3.19 that the majority of first consultations took place at the client's home in both Lewisham and Deptford and in the local GP practice in Ashford.

Table 3.21 shows the proportion of second and subsequent consultations that took place in different locations. It indicates that these were mostly provided in the local community, especially in the client's own home and local GP practices. There was a very high proportion of home-based consultations in Lewisham, with over three-quarters of all second and subsequent consultations (76 per cent) taking place in the client's home, and almost as many in Deptford (68 per cent). In Ashford the picture was completely different, as only one third of second and subsequent consultations took place at home (34 per cent) compared with 64 per cent at the woman's local GP practice. In Lewisham nearly one fifth of second and subsequent consultations (19 per cent) were held at the GP practice. The absence of any significant links between the Deptford MGP and local GPs can be seen by the fact that only *one* consultation was held at a GP practice.

Table 3.21 Location of second and subsequent consultations with women

column percentages

	Lewisham	Ashford	Deptford
Client's home	76	34	66
GP surgery	19	64	*
Hospital	5	2	7
Relative's/Partner's/ Friend's home	*	*	2
Midwife's home	0	0	2
Albany Centre	0	0	19
Client's workplace	*	0	0
More than one location	*	*	2
n.a.	*	*	2
Base: all second and subsequent consultations	*(3,098)*	*(2,765)*	*(900)*

Hospital consultations (at an antenatal clinic, day assessment or foetal assessment unit, labour ward, ultrasound department or hospital ward) were much more likely to occur in Deptford (7 per cent) than Lewisham (5 per cent) or Ashford (2 per cent). Another 2 per cent of all the second and subsequent consultations in Deptford occurred in more than one location, usually starting at home and then proceeding to the hospital. The higher proportion of hospital consultations recorded in Deptford is largely attributable to the fact that these women were more likely than those in other areas to be accompanied by their midwife to specialist consultations.

The figures clearly show that the MGPs were highly successful in providing community-based antenatal consultations (booking and subsequent consultations). The provision of readily and easily accessible antenatal care was organised primarily around the GP practices in Ashford compared with the client's own home in Lewisham and Deptford. The implications of concentrating resources in different locations are discussed in Appendix D.

Continuity of antenatal care and number of consultations

Changing Childbirth discusses the value placed on trusted and familiar faces by women at critical points in pregnancy and childbirth, such as when complications arose or when they went into labour. Women also emphasised the importance of having professionals who were aware of their history, plans and preferences.

The MGPs sought to ensure continuity of care by assigning a named midwife to care for and support each woman throughout pregnancy and, where possible, to attend the birth. In Deptford women were booked by two midwives, one acting as a primary midwife and the other as a secondary midwife.

In order to determine whether women saw the same midwife throughout pregnancy the name of the midwife seen at each second and subsequent consultation was recorded. We looked at the number of second and subsequent consultations where women saw their named midwife as a proportion of the total number of MGP consultations.

It should be noted that Table 3.22 includes information on the mean number of second and subsequent consultations by each MGP as well as those carried out by the named midwife. The table shows that a very high proportion of MGP consultations were carried out by the named midwife for all women who had one or more second and subsequent consultations in Ashford (92 per cent) and Lewisham (87 per cent). The lower figure in Deptford (68 per cent) may be attributed to the fact that women were cared for by a pair of midwives and only the primary midwife could be included in the analysis.

Table 3.22 **Proportion of second and subsequent consultations carried out by named midwife in each MGP**

column percentages

	Lewisham	Ashford	Deptford
Named midwife consultations	87	92	68
Other MGP MW	13	8	32
Mean number of MGP second and subsequent consultations	7.2	5.9	6.1
Mean number of named MW second and subsequent consultations	6.3	5.5	4.4
Base: all second and subsequent consultations	*(3,098)*	*(2,765)*	*(900)*

The extent to which continuity of care was achieved by individual midwives in each of the MGPs was analysed by looking at the proportion of second and subsequent consultations carried out by individual midwives in the three areas for women on their caseload and the number of visits carried out by other midwives.

• In Lewisham the proportion of second and subsequent consultations carried out by individual midwives for women on their own caseloads ranged from 83 per cent to 93 per cent. If consultations were carried out by other midwives they were usually midwives based at the same GP practice as the named midwife.

• In Ashford 88 to 99 per cent of all the consultations carried out by midwives were for women on their own caseloads.

• The number of consultations carried out by individual midwives for women on their own caseload in Deptford ranged from 63 per cent to 87 per cent. Although it is likely that a certain proportion of the visits were carried out by the secondary midwife, the flexible rather than fixed partnership arrangement in Deptford makes a clearer picture of antenatal continuity of carer more difficult to determine.

Working with other professionals

Changing Childbirth discusses the role of key professionals such as midwives, GPs, obstetricians and junior hospital doctors, outlining the importance of working in partnership in the best interests of women. It is clear that a partnership arrangement in the provision of maternity care should develop from a mutual understanding of what each professional can contribute, and an acceptance of the view that the best results are often achieved by including rather than excluding other professionals. These issues played an important role in this evaluation and are discussed in the final chapter.

Referrals to a consultant obstetrician at the first consultation with the MGP

We asked midwives to record whether women were referred to a consultant obstetrician at their first consultation and the reason for the referral. Over a quarter of the women in Ashford (26 per cent) were referred to a consultant obstetrician at the first consultation, compared with Lewisham (12 per cent) and Deptford where only 5 per cent of women were referred. The referral rate in Ashford is roughly similar to the proportion of women who chose or were assigned a consultant obstetrician as their lead professional at their first visit.

Referrals in all areas were most often triggered by a discussion about obstetric/medical history or current problems experienced in pregnancy. Only 8 women altogether were referred to a consultant in Deptford, mainly because of current or previous problems in pregnancy. It should be remembered that over 40 per cent of women in Deptford had already received care elsewhere and may have seen a consultant before transferring to the Deptford MGP. Of the women referred to a consultant, in 70 per cent of cases in Ashford and 65 per cent in Lewisham, it was because of a previous obstetric or medical history. Women in Ashford were much more likely to have requested a referral (21 per cent) than women in Deptford and Lewisham. A handful of women in all areas were referred to discuss prenatal tests.

Referrals to a consultant obstetrician during second and subsequent consultations

Referrals to a consultant obstetrician were made at 4 per cent of the second and subsequent consultations in Ashford compared with 8 per cent in Deptford and 7 per cent in Lewisham. A higher proportion of referrals to obstetricians in Deptford were requested by women themselves compared with Ashford and, surprisingly, no women in Lewisham were recorded as requesting a referral.

Most of the referrals at second and subsequent consultations made by the Deptford MGP were to consultant obstetricians at King's College Hospital, around one in six to Lewisham Hospital, one in ten to Guy's Hospital and the remainder to Greenwich Hospital.

Nearly all the referrals in Ashford were made to consultant obstetricians in William Harvey Hospital, with around a half of the referrals made to one consultant, a quarter to a second consultant, one in ten to a third consultant and only a handful to a fourth consultant. A few referrals were sent to unspecified consultants at King's College Hospital.

In Lewisham the same picture emerged, with most referrals directed to consultant obstetricians in Lewisham Hospital. Over one third of the referrals went to one consultant, less than one quarter to a second consultant, less than one fifth to a third consultant and one in ten to a fourth consultant. Some referrals were also directed to obstetric registrars, to Guy's Hospital and to Farnborough Hospital.

Specific problems or complications in the woman's current pregnancy or a previous obstetric history of note were the most common reasons for referrals in Ashford (79 per cent) and Deptford (60 per cent) and accounted for 38 per cent of the referrals in Lewisham. However, the most common reason cited in Lewisham (40 per cent) was to request an induction date for women who were post term, compared with 10 per cent of the referrals in Ashford and only one woman in Deptford. In fact, a higher proportion of women in Deptford actually delivered at 41 and 42 weeks in Deptford than elsewhere but midwives were less likely to make a referral for this reason. The remainder of referrals to consultants requested a review and assessment of options and choices for care in pregnancy for women who had a previous medical or obstetric history or who had particular social problems.

Referrals to a GP at the first consultation with the MGP

The big difference between Deptford and the other areas was the absence of referrals to GPs at the first consultation. Referring women to GPs in Ashford was more common practice than elsewhere. Only 4 per cent of the women in Deptford were referred to their GP at the first consultation compared with nearly two-thirds of women in Ashford (61 per cent) and over one third of women in Lewisham (36 per cent). A quarter of all the referrals in Lewisham occurred at the GP's request. However, the most common reason cited for referral in all areas was for a physical examination. Only a handful of women were referred to a GP at their own request and none of the women in Deptford asked to be referred to their GP at all. The figures show that GPs in Deptford were less likely to have been involved in women's care, and the continued lack of referrals to GPs during second and subsequent consultations reinforces this point.

Referrals to a GP during second and subsequent consultations

Referrals to GPs during second and subsequent consultations were relatively uncommon in all areas but especially in Deptford. Referrals to GPs were made at 6 per cent of the second and subsequent consultations with women in Lewisham and Ashford and at only 3 per cent of consultations in Deptford, reinforcing the view that the GPs had a peripheral role in the provision of antenatal care.

In Lewisham just under half of the referrals were at the GP's request, indicating that they had taken measures to ensure that they would remain involved in women's care and usually requested to see women twice during pregnancy. 16 per cent of referrals were for specific non-pregnancy related health problems, 20 per cent were for pregnancy related health problems or complications that required medical advice or attention. A few women were referred to their GP to request a prescription.

In Ashford 16 per cent of referrals were for non-pregnancy related health problems and nearly a quarter were for specific pregnancy related health problems or complications. Over a quarter of women were referred for a prescription, and 14 per cent were referred for a physical examination at some point in pregnancy, often at the GP's request.

Referrals to a GP in Deptford were most often made for a prescription or for advice on pregnancy related or non-pregnancy related health problems.

Chapter 4

Labour, delivery and the postnatal period

Following the discussion of antenatal care in Chapter 3, this chapter looks at the outcomes for all women who had booked with the midwifery group practices (MGPs) during the monitoring period 1 April 1994 to 30 September 1995. Intrapartum and postnatal care will also be discussed with reference, where appropriate, to the preferences and choices expressed by women at their first consultation with the MGPs. At the end of this chapter we look at continuity of care for all women who were delivered by the MGPs during the monitoring period, including those who had booked with the midwives before the monitoring period started in April 1994. Details of these deliveries were given in Table 3.5 in Chapter 3.

Outcome of pregnancy of women who booked during monitoring period

Outcome details were submitted by the midwives for over two-thirds of the women who had booked with the Lewisham and Deptford MGPs and 61 per cent of women who had booked with the Ashford MGP during the monitoring period April 1994 to September 1995. In addition, 'transfer of care' forms were submitted for 13 per cent of all women booking with the Ashford MGP, confirming that their care had been taken over by the JACANES II group of midwives because they fulfilled the criteria for consultant-led care. Midwives were asked to record the outcome of each pregnancy and Table 4.1 shows the proportion of outcomes under different category headings.

91 per cent of the outcomes in Lewisham, 88 per cent in Deptford and 85 per cent in Ashford related to maternities. The remainder of the outcomes in all areas were confirmation of miscarriages, missed abortions, termination of pregnancy, or movement by the client away from MGP care or out of the area. One of the differences between Ashford and the other MGPs was the higher rate of miscarriage (7 per cent), compared with

Lewisham (3 per cent) and Deptford (4 per cent) which could, it appeared, be attributed in part to the Ashford system of early bookings.

Table 4.1   Outcome of pregnancy for women booking with the MGPs

column percentages

	Lewisham	Ashford	Deptford
Outcome			
Baby alive at discharge from midwife	91	85	88
Born alive but died before discharge	*	*	2
Stillbirth	*	*	1
Miscarriage	3	7	4
Missed abortion	0	*	)
Termination of pregnancy	1	1	1
Client moved	5	6	4
n.a.	0	*	1
Base: all women with outcome details	*(345)*	*(337)*	*(113)*

* equals less than 1 per cent

Number of weeks gestation at delivery

Table 4.2 shows that a relatively small proportion of women in the three areas had pre-term deliveries, but this was slightly higher for women in Lewisham (6 per cent) and Ashford (7 per cent) than in Deptford (3 per cent). 35 to 40 per cent of women in all areas delivered between 37 and 39 weeks gestation. Around one third of women in Lewisham and Ashford delivered at 40 weeks compared with over a quarter in Deptford. Women in Deptford were more likely to deliver at 41 or 42 weeks (30 per cent) compared with a quarter of women in Lewisham and over one fifth of women in Ashford, which is important to note given the number of women who transferred to the Deptford MGP after 31 and even after 36 weeks gestation.

Sex and birthweight of live babies

In Lewisham 50 per cent of the babies were male and 49 per cent were female. Details of the sex of the baby was not available in 1 per cent of cases, mostly because deliveries had taken place in other hospitals. The same proportion of male babies (54 per cent) and female babies (46 per cent) were born in Ashford and Deptford.

Table 4.2   Number of weeks gestation at delivery

column percentages

	Lewisham	Ashford	Deptford
36 weeks and under	6	7	3
37 weeks	4	5	7
38 weeks	12	16	7
39 weeks	19	19	25
40 weeks	32	31	27
41 weeks	19	16	22
42 weeks	6	6	8
n.a.	2	0	2
Mean number of weeks gestation	*39.4*	*39.0*	*39.6*
Base: all maternities except stillbirths	*(314)*	*(287)*	*(102*

In Lewisham the average birthweight of live singleton babies was slightly lower (3366.5 grams) than in Ashford (3411.2 grams) and Deptford (3477.2 grams). The average birthweight of twin babies was 2766.6 grams in Lewisham and 1860 grams in Ashford. No twins were born in Deptford.

Duration of labour

The average length of labour for women in Ashford was shorter (7.88 hours) than for women in Lewisham (9.01 hours) and Deptford (9.99 hours). (The length of labour should be related to parity.)

Mode of delivery

Table 4.3 shows the proportion of women in each area who had a normal vaginal delivery, instrumental delivery or a caesarean section. A high proportion of women in all areas had a normal vaginal delivery but the data do not indicate whether the vaginal deliveries were spontaneous or induced. 82 per cent of women in Lewisham had a normal vaginal delivery compared with 79 per cent in Ashford and Deptford. Women in Ashford and Deptford were less likely to have had an instrumental delivery (6 per cent in both areas) than in Lewisham (9 per cent), but were also more likely to have had a caesarean section (16 and 15 per cent respectively) than women in Lewisham (9 per cent).

The caesarean section rate in Ashford is notably high, if one takes into account that 13 per cent of all the women who had booked with the MGP were *transferred out of the evaluation before they delivered* because they were deemed to be high risk and satisfied the eligibility criteria for consultant-led care.

A very small proportion of women in Deptford who had a vaginal or instrumental delivery had an episiotomy (5 per cent), compared with over a quarter of women in Ashford and less than one fifth in Lewisham. Around a third of women in all areas who had a normal vaginal or instrumental delivery sustained a tear during labour. However, the data do not indicate the degree of the tear or whether suturing had been carried out.

Table 4.3   Mode of delivery for all maternities

			column percentages
	Lewisham	Ashford	Deptford
Vaginal	82	79	79
Instrumental	9	6	6
Caesarean	9	16	15
Base: all maternities except stillbirths	*(314)*	*(287)*	*(102)*

Continuity of intrapartum care

Presence of named midwife during first stage labour and delivery

One of the key objectives of *Changing Childbirth* was that 75 per cent of women should be cared for in labour by a midwife whom they had come to know. We have already seen that a very high proportion of women were offered a choice of lead professional (or had already chosen) and that the majority of women in all areas opted for midwife-led care. In addition, where an MGP midwife was not the lead professional, women were still assigned a named midwife who provided their care during pregnancy. The MGPs also placed emphasis on the fact that should the named midwife not be available at any point during pregnancy or when the woman went into labour, she would, as far as possible, be cared for by another MGP midwife. Women were regularly invited to meet all the MGP midwives so that they could become familiar with the group. Deptford was different again in that each woman was cared for by a partnership of two midwives, with one taking a primary midwife role and another taking a secondary midwife role.

We asked the midwives to record whether the woman was attended at first stage labour and delivery by her named midwife and to record if other MGP midwives or hospital midwives were present. Table 4.4 indicates that women in Deptford were twice as likely to have their named or primary midwife attend them in first stage labour and at delivery than women in Ashford. This undoubtedly reflects the much smaller caseloads of the Deptford midwives. The difference between Deptford and Lewisham was not as marked.

Table 4.4   Presence of named midwife, other MGP midwife, hospital and student midwife during first stage labour and delivery

column percentages

	First stage labour			Delivery		
	Lew	Ash	Dept	Lew	Ash	Dept
Midwife present						
Named MW only	38	21	19	32	23	17
Named MW plus one other MGP MW	10	14	66	13	9	75
Named MW plus two or more MGP MWs	1	6	2	*	1	0
Named MW plus hospital MW	5	4	1	12	5	3
Named MW plus Student MW	3	2	2	4	4	0
Other MGP MW	26	13	1	25	21	1
Two or more MGP MWs	2	6	2	2	4	2
Other MGP MW plus hospital MW/student MW	*	1	0	4	1	0
Hospital MWs/student MW	5	21	0	6	30	1
No labour	4	9	6	0	0	0
n.a.	5	2	1	2	*	0
Base: all maternities except stillbirths	*(314)*	*(287)*	*(102)*	*(314)*	*(287)*	*(102)*

Deptford

93 per cent of women in Deptford were attended in first stage *labour* by their primary or another MGP midwife. However, it is necessary to look at how this figure breaks down in order to draw some conclusions about the resourcing implications of providing intrapartum continuity of care. A key difference between Deptford and elsewhere was that 90 per cent of Deptford women were attended during first stage labour by their primary midwife. Looking at this in more detail:

• 19 per cent of women were attended by their primary midwife only

- 66 per cent by the primary midwife and one other MGP midwife
- 2 per cent by the primary and two other MGP midwives
- 1 per cent by the primary midwife and a hospital midwife
- 2 per cent by the primary midwife and a student or placement midwife
- 3 per cent were attended by another MGP midwife in the absence of the primary midwife.

98 per cent of women were attended during *delivery* by their primary or another MGP midwife, with as many as 95 per cent attended by their primary midwife:

- 17 per cent of women were attended by the primary midwife alone
- 75 per cent by the primary midwife and another MGP midwife
- 3 per cent by the primary midwife and a hospital midwife
- 3 per cent of women by another MGP midwife in the absence of the primary midwife.

Lewisham

In Lewisham 85 per cent of women were attended in first stage *labour* by the named midwife or another MGP midwife. Looking at this further, 57 per cent were attended during the first stage of labour by their named midwife:

- 38 per cent of women were attended by the named midwife only
- 11 per cent by the named and another MGP midwife
- 5 per cent by the named midwife and a hospital midwife
- 3 per cent by the named midwife and a student midwife
- 28 per cent of women were attended by an MGP midwife in the absence of the named midwife.

92 per cent of women were attended by their named midwife or an MGP midwife during the actual *delivery*, with 61 per cent attended by their named midwife:

- 32 per cent were attended by their named midwife only
- 13 per cent by the named midwife plus one other MGP midwife
- 12 per cent by the named midwife and a hospital midwife
- 4 per cent by the named and a student midwife
- 31 per cent of women were attended by another MGP midwife in the absence of the named midwife.

These Lewisham figures for named midwives are very high when the total number of women delivering during the monitoring period is taken into account, but the question of whether this level of activity can be sustained in the longer term will be discussed later.

Ashford

Over two-thirds of women (67 per cent) in Ashford were attended in first stage *labour* by their named or another MGP midwife. Women were less likely to have their named midwife present during first stage labour than elsewhere (47 per cent):

- 21 per cent were attended by their named midwife only
- 14 per cent by the named midwife and one other MGP midwife
- 6 per cent by the named midwife and two other MGP midwives
- 4 per cent by the named midwife and a hospital midwife
- 2 per cent by the named midwife and a student midwife
- 20 per cent were attended by an MGP midwife in the absence of the named midwife .

68 per cent of women were attended at *delivery* by their named midwife or another MGP midwife, with 42 per cent attended by their named midwife:

- 23 per cent were attended by their named midwife only
- 9 per cent by the named and one other MGP midwife
- 1 per cent by the named midwife and two MGP midwives
- 5 per cent by the named midwife and a hospital midwife
- 4 per cent by the named midwife and a student midwife
- 26 per cent by another MGP midwife in the absence of the named midwife.

The remainder of the women were attended at delivery by hospital midwives, underlining the fact that the Ashford MGP were giving antenatal care in the first twelve months of the monitoring period to women who were unlikely to have been delivered by them, given the fact that they were receiving consultant obstetrician-led care.

The provision of intrapartum continuity of care in light of the actual workload and caseloads of the MGPs will be discussed at the end of this chapter.

Why was the named midwife not present during the birth?

The most common reason cited for the absence of the named midwife was because she was off duty, on annual leave or sick leave. This occurred more often in Lewisham (72 per cent of cases where the named midwife was not present) than in Ashford (53 per cent), and accounted for most of the non-attendance in Deptford where only 5 cases were cited overall. Another reason cited in Lewisham (11 per cent) and Ashford (6 per cent) was because the woman was booked to deliver at another hospital. In a few cases the midwife was called too late, usually by the client because of the unexpected or rapid progress of labour. In a handful of other cases the midwife was attending another woman or the hospital staff failed to call or inform the MGP midwife on time.

15 per cent of women in Ashford who did not have a named midwife present at the birth were booked for consultant care from the outset and another 15 per cent were transferred to consultant care because of complications during pregnancy or during labour.

Time spent with women in labour

We have already seen that women in Deptford had a slightly longer labour (9.99 hours) than women in Lewisham (9.01 hours) and women in Ashford (7.88 hours). Midwives were asked to record the length of time the woman was attended in labour when the named midwife was present. This information was supplied for 57 per cent of the births in Lewisham, 47 per cent in Ashford and 90 per cent in Deptford.

The figures show that the named midwife in Ashford spent on average the least time with women in labour (5.95 hours), probably because the duration of labour was shorter for women in Ashford than elsewhere. In Deptford the named or primary midwife spent on average 7.8 hours with women in labour while in Lewisham the average was 8.07 hours. In both Lewisham and Ashford the named midwife spent more time with women when alone than when another midwife was also present. We found the reverse to be true in Deptford: that is, midwives spent less time with women when alone and more time when another midwife was present.

Where did women deliver and was this in the booked location?

We have already seen that women in Deptford were more likely to opt for a home birth than elsewhere and that hospital births were chosen by the majority of women in Lewisham and Ashford. Table 4.5 shows that nearly two-thirds of the women in Deptford (63 per cent) had a home birth, compared with 16 per cent in Lewisham and 7 per cent in Ashford. Ashford had the highest proportion of hospital births (93 per cent) compared with Lewisham (84 per cent) and Deptford (37 per cent).

Table 4.5   Location of delivery

column percentages

	Lewisham	Ashford	Deptford
Location			
Home	16	7	63
Hospital	84	93	37
Base: all maternities except stillbirths	*(314)*	*(287)*	*(102)*

Midwives were asked to record whether the delivery had taken place in the booked location. 89 per cent of women in Ashford delivered in the booked location, compared with 85 per cent of women in Lewisham and 70 per cent of women in Deptford.

- In *Ashford,* 93 per cent of the women delivering in hospital appeared to have planned to do so at the first consultation while in 3 per cent of cases it was not clear whether the hospital birth was planned or not. 4 per cent of the women who delivered in hospital (11 women) had originally opted for a home birth: 6 women subsequently changed their minds and 5 women had to have a hospital birth because of complications that made a home birth unfeasible.

  8 of the 19 women who had a home birth appeared to have planned this at booking, 5 women opted for a home birth at some point during pregnancy and one decided to have a home birth during labour. The remaining 5 women had an unplanned home birth because of their rapid progress during labour.

- In *Lewisham,* 93 per cent of women who delivered in hospital had chosen this at the first consultation. In 2 per cent of cases it was not clear if the hospital birth was planned from booking. 3 per cent had opted for a home birth but delivered in hospital because of complications that arose either during pregnancy or labour, or because an induction of labour was recommended, and 2 per cent of women changed their minds from a home to a hospital birth during pregnancy.

  Over half of the women who delivered at home (26 women) had planned to do so from the outset. 14 per cent of all the home births were unplanned (7 women) and occurred because of the rapid progress of labour. 9 women decided to have a home birth during their pregnancy and 4 women opted to have a home birth just before or during labour.

- Over 80 per cent of the home births in *Deptford* (52 home births) had been planned from the booking consultation. In three cases the woman opted for a home birth during pregnancy and in three cases during the actual labour. Two women appeared to have had an unplanned home birth due to the rapid progress of labour and in four cases it was not clear if the home birth was planned or unplanned.

  Over half of the hospital births (22 hospital births) were planned from the outset. 13 of the women who delivered in hospital had originally opted for a home birth but did not have one because of complications that arose during pregnancy (3 cases) or during labour (10 cases). A further 3 women who delivered in hospital had also originally opted for a home birth but changed their minds during pregnancy.

The figures clearly show that if hospital was the preferred place of delivery women would nearly always deliver there unless they had an unexpectedly quick labour and thereby had an unplanned home birth. However, if a home birth was chosen, women were less likely to deliver in their preferred location. This underlines the importance of discussing the possibility of having to opt for a hospital birth at some stage in pregnancy or even during labour itself. In terms of outcome, it is interesting to look at the proportion of women in Ashford and Lewisham who had unplanned home births and the proportion of women in Deptford who had planned home births but had a hospital birth.

Doctors present at first stage labour and delivery

a) Consultant obstetrician

We asked midwives to record on all outcome forms whether a consultant obstetrician was present at labour (first stage) and delivery. The figures demonstrate that the presence of a consultant obstetrician at any stage during birth was uncommon in all areas and especially in Lewisham where a consultant was present on only a handful of occasions: for 2 per cent of women during labour and 1 per cent at delivery. In Ashford a consultant was present for 5 per cent of women during labour and 3 per cent at delivery while in Deptford a consultant was present at 5 per cent of labours and deliveries. On more than half of the occasions when a consultant was present this was because a labour ward round was being held, while in the remainder of cases the consultant attended to advise on the management of specific problems or complications.

b) Other doctors present

Table 4.6 shows the proportion of women who were attended by doctors other than consultant obstetricians at first stage labour and/or delivery. Table 4.6 shows that, although women in Deptford were less likely to have a doctor present during birth than elsewhere, most of the women who delivered in hospital were attended at some stage by a doctor. Most doctors attending women at birth were hospital doctors and only a few women were attended by a GP. 37 per cent of *all* births in Deptford were in hospital and 34 per cent of all Deptford women were attended at some stage by a doctor, in almost all cases a hospital doctor.

In contrast, 93 per cent of all births in Ashford and 84 per cent in Lewisham were in hospital and around a half of *all* women in both areas had a doctor present. 20 per cent of women in Deptford and Ashford had doctors present at both labour and delivery compared with 13 per cent of women in Lewisham. However, a higher proportion of women in Lewisham had doctor/s present at labour or delivery than elsewhere.

Table 4.6   Women attended by doctors during labour and/or delivery

column percentages

	Lewisham	Ashford	Deptford
None	49	53	66
Labour only	19	14	6
Delivery only	16	13	8
Both labour and delivery	13	19	20
n.a.	3	1	0
Base: all maternities			
except stillbirths	*(314)*	*(287)*	*(102)*

Doctors present during the first stage of labour

Nearly three-quarters of the women in Lewisham (73 per cent) who were attended by a doctor in first stage labour went on to have a normal vaginal delivery compared with 67 per cent in Ashford and 48 per cent in Deptford. Doctors more commonly attended women in labour to review their progress or to give advice and manage complications detected before or during labour. Other reasons cited were to site an intravenous cannula, epidural cannula or to prescribe drugs.

A higher proportion of women in Deptford were attended by a registrar (78 per cent) than in Ashford (65 per cent) and Lewisham (48 per cent). Around half of the women in all areas were attended by an SHO in labour. Only a few women had a GP or paediatrician present. Over a quarter of women in Lewisham had an anaesthetist present compared with a fifth of women in both Ashford and Deptford.

Doctors present during the delivery

The most common reasons cited for doctors being present during the actual delivery were to perform a caesarean section or an instrumental delivery and some doctors, especially registrars and senior house officers (SHOs), had also been present at first stage labour to review progress and manage complications. 69 per cent of women attended by a doctor during delivery in Deptford, 66 per cent in Ashford and 57 per cent in Lewisham had an instrumental delivery or caesarean section carried out.

75 per cent of women in Ashford were attended during delivery by a registrar compared with around two-thirds of women in Deptford (65 per cent) and 57 per cent of women in Lewisham. Two-thirds of women in Deptford (65 per cent) were attended by an SHO, 43 per cent in Ashford and 38 per cent in Lewisham. As expected, a higher proportion of paediatricians were in attendance at delivery than during first stage labour. A

higher proportion of anaesthetists were also present during delivery in Ashford and Deptford.

Who else was present at first stage labour and delivery?

Women in Deptford were much more likely to say they wanted their partner and family around them when labour preferences were discussed at the first consultation. 20 per cent of the women who had expressed labour preferences emphasised having family around but this was not mentioned to the same extent by women in Lewisham or Ashford.

A very high proportion of close relatives and friends were present with women during the first stage of labour and delivery. 89 per cent of women in all areas had their husband, partner, boyfriend or father of the baby present with them during the first stage of labour. A slightly lower proportion were present at the delivery: 86 per cent in Ashford and Deptford and 87 per cent in Lewisham.

Women in Lewisham and Deptford were twice as likely to have relatives present during labour and delivery than women in Ashford (14 per cent). A major difference between Deptford and elsewhere was the high proportion of women who had friends present during labour (24 per cent) and delivery (23 per cent), compared with Lewisham where 8 per cent of women had friends present during labour and 6 per cent at the delivery. In Ashford women were least likely to have had friends present during labour (2 per cent) or delivery (2 per cent).

What form of pain control did women use in labour?

We have seen that pain control was important to women in Ashford and Lewisham who had expressed labour preferences at their first consultation, while for some women in Deptford a preference for minimal or no analgesia was often expressed. We asked midwives to record the pain relief agents used by women during labour. Table 4.7 shows the type of pain relief agents used by women in each area by the location of delivery. Women who did not go through the first stage of labour are presented separately in the table.

This table shows that in all areas women who delivered at home were far less likely to have used any pain relief agents, especially in Deptford and Ashford. Less than half of the women who had had a home birth in Ashford and Deptford used pain relief compared with two-thirds in Lewisham. Entonox and TENS were the most common pain relief agents used by women delivering at home in Lewisham and Ashford, while water and Entonox were most commonly used by women who had home births in Deptford. Unrestricted mobility as a pain relief option was also used by a few women in Deptford.

Table 4.7   Pain control used in labour by location of delivery

column percentages

| | Hospital | | | Home | | |
	Lew	Ash	Dept	Lew	Ash	Dept
None	8	11	13	31	53	59
Epidural	21	15	39	0	0	0
Entonox	70	55	45	61	21	17
Pethidine	28	32	0	0	0	0
TENS	11	13	3	27	26	5
Water	*	3	21	2	5	27
Massage	*	*	3	0	0	0
Aromatherapy	0	*	0	2	0	0
Unrestricted mobility	-	*	0	0	0	0
General anaesthetic	*	3	3	0	0	0
No labour	5	10	16	0	0	0
n.a.	*	*	3	0	0	0
Base: all maternities in hospital and at home	*(265)*	*(268)*	*(38)*	*(49)*	*(19)*	*(64)*

Percentages add to more than 100 per cent because women used more than one method of pain control.

Women in Lewisham and Ashford who delivered in hospital were more likely to use narcotic pain relief than women in Deptford. Pethidine was used by 32 per cent of women who delivered in hospital in Ashford, 28 per cent of women in Lewisham and by none of the women in Deptford who delivered in hospital. Entonox was the most common pain relief agent used by women in all areas. In Deptford 39 per cent of women who delivered in hospital had an epidural compared with 21 per cent in Lewisham and 15 per cent in Ashford. Water was used as a pain relief agent by 21 per cent of women in Deptford, 3 per cent in Ashford and by only a tiny number of women in Lewisham.

Overall, a higher proportion of women in Deptford did not use any pain relief agents or were more likely to use non-pharmacological pain relief agents than women elsewhere. As might be expected, there were clear differences in the type of pain relief agents used by women delivering at home and in hospital across all areas, with a greater proportion of women opting for pharmacological pain relief agents in hospital.

Length of hospital stay

We have already seen that 93 per cent of women delivered at hospital in Ashford, 84 per cent in Lewisham and 37 per cent in Deptford. We have also seen how attractive DOMINO delivery was to women who chose to deliver their baby at hospital. For instance, 70 per cent of the women who were offered a choice of place of birth chose a DOMINO delivery in Ashford compared to over half in Lewisham and just over one fifth in Deptford. We asked midwives to record the length of the woman's stay at hospital on the outcome forms to determine whether women had the short hospital stay that many wished to have.

Table 4.8 shows that women in Deptford were more likely to have a shorter hospital stay (an average of 2.3 days) than women in Lewisham (3.1 days) or women in Ashford (3.6 days). It is interesting that in Deptford this short hospital stay coincided with the highest proportion of caesarean sections. 39 per cent of the Deptford women who delivered in hospital had a caesarean section, compared with 17 per cent in Ashford and 11 per cent in Lewisham.

Table 4.8   Length of hospital stay for women who delivered in hospital

column percentages

	Lewisham	Ashford	Deptford
Same day discharge	13	9	34
1 day	25	19	16
2 days	19	19	16
3 days	14	11	8
4 plus days	26	35	24
n.a.	3	1	5
Mean stay in days	*3.1*	*3.6*	*2.3*
Base: all women who delivered in hospital	*(265)*	*(268)*	*(38)*

47 per cent of the women in Deptford who delivered in hospital were discharged on the same day as their admission or on the next day, compared with 38 per cent of women in Lewisham and 34 per cent in Ashford. Overall, nearly three-quarters of all the women who delivered in hospital in Lewisham and Deptford (71 per cent) were discharged up to three days after admission compared with 64 per cent of the women in Ashford. 35 per cent of women in Ashford, 26 per cent in Lewisham and 24 per cent in Deptford were discharged from hospital on or after 4 days. (These figures relate to the overall length of hospital stay, not hospital stay post delivery.)

Length of hospital stay has often been taken as an outcome measure which enables certain judgements to be made about the effectiveness of care. In addition, there are cost savings and financial benefits for hospitals if a quick throughput of women is achieved. However, shorter hospital stays should not necessarily be taken as a positive sign unless women favourably endorse the quality of the care received during their stay. Some of our interviews with women revealed that they sought to go home before they felt they were able and ready to do so because they were not satisfied with their care in hospital. This shows that an analysis of length of hospital stay in itself is not sufficient and should be related to women's perception of the quality of care they received as in-patients.

In order to determine the proportion of women in each area who actually had a DOMINO delivery we have taken same day and next day discharge as the nearest estimate possible. Next day discharge is included because some women may have delivered late on the previous night and although this makes the time-frame rather broad it still provides an estimate of DOMINO deliveries. Looking at the date of delivery and date of discharge we found that Deptford women were more likely to have had a DOMINO delivery than elsewhere.

Postnatal consultations and continuity of postnatal care

In discussing the organisation and provision of postnatal care, *Changing Childbirth* emphasises the importance of a flexible approach agreed in conjunction with each woman to ensure that her different needs and support requirements are met.

Midwives were asked to record the total number of postnatal consultations that each woman received and to indicate the number of consultations provided by the named and other MGP midwives, as well as the number provided by hospital and other community midwives. The average number of postnatal visits by all professionals including MGP midwives, hospital midwives and other community midwives was highest in Lewisham where women received on average 11 visits compared with 8.5 in Ashford and 9.1 in Deptford.

However, women in Deptford received a higher proportion of postnatal visits from MGP midwives than in either Ashford or Lewisham. 92 per cent of all the postnatal consultations carried out in Deptford were by MGP midwives, 7 per cent by hospital midwives and 1 per cent by community midwives. This is likely to result from the fact that Deptford also had a higher proportion of home births so that many women did not receive postnatal care from hospital or other community midwives.

85 per cent of all postnatal consultations recorded in Lewisham were carried out by MGP midwives, 15 per cent by hospital midwives and less than 1 per cent by other community midwives. The Lewisham MGP tended to initiate MGP postnatal care while women were still in hospital which maximised the MGP's overall input and reduced the input from hospital midwives. In Ashford around two-thirds of postnatal consultations were carried out by MGP midwives (64 per cent), over one third by hospital midwives (35 per cent) and 1 per cent by other community midwives.

Were women cared for postnatally by their named midwife?

In order to determine whether women had received continuity of postnatal care we looked at the number and breakdown of MGP postnatal consultations for each area. Table 4.9 indicates that all of the MGPs succeeded in providing continuity of postnatal care. However, as it was not possible to tell whether women saw the same hospital or community midwife, an overall impression of continuity is more difficult to assess. The average number of MGP postnatal consultations was higher for Lewisham and Deptford (9.2 and 8.8 visits) than Ashford (5.4 visits).

Table 4.9   Proportion of postnatal consultations carried out by the named and other MGP midwives

column percentages

	Lewisham	Ashford	Deptford
Named midwife	73	77	71
Second midwife	22	20	28
Third midwife	4	3	2
Fourth midwife	*	*	0
Mean number of consultations with an MGP MW	9.2	5.4	8.8
Base: all MGP postnatal consultations	(2,878)	(1,565)	(895)

- 95 per cent of all MGP postnatal consultations involved the named or one other midwife in *Lewisham*. The named midwife accounted for just under three-quarters of the MGP postnatal consultations, a second MGP midwife accounted for 22 per cent, a third midwife for 4 per cent, and a fourth midwife for less than 1 per cent of MGP consultations.

- 97 per cent of all MGP postnatal consultations were carried out by the named midwife or one other MGP midwife in *Ashford*. The named midwife alone accounted for 77 per cent of the MGP consultations, a second MGP midwife accounted for one fifth, a third midwife for 3 per cent, and a fourth midwife carried out less than 1 per cent of MGP consultations.

- In *Deptford*, 99 per cent of all MGP postnatal consultations were carried out by the named (primary) or one other MGP midwife. The named midwife accounted for 71 per cent of the MGP visits, a second MGP midwife accounted for 28 per cent and a third midwife for 2 per cent of MGP consultations.

Did mother or baby experience any health problems before being discharged from their named midwife?

Morbidity has become increasingly important as a predictor of the quality and effectiveness of maternity care. We asked midwives to record any health problems experienced by women and their babies between delivery and discharge from their named midwife.

a) Problems experienced by women

32 per cent of women in Deptford were recorded as experiencing notable health problems compared with 18 per cent of women in Lewisham and 19 per cent in Ashford. Some were minor health problems but nonetheless caused some distress and discomfort to women, while others were more severe complications requiring medical attention and intervention. These included postpartum haemorrhage, retention of the placenta and thrombosis. Much depended, of course, on how the midwives interpreted 'health problems'. Complications were more prevalent in Ashford (35 per cent of those reporting health problems) and Lewisham (28 per cent) than in Deptford (12 per cent).

Difficulties associated with breast feeding such as sore breasts and nipples or more severe problems such as mastitis were experienced by over half the women with health problems in Deptford and only one fifth in Lewisham and Ashford. Some women experienced minor unrelated health problems such as colds and flu, while others experienced a recurrence or exacerbation of long-standing medical problems. Both were more commonly reported in Lewisham and Deptford than in Ashford. A handful of women in all areas had experienced a period of 'postnatal blues', some of whom had had previous problems with postnatal blues or depression.

More women in Ashford who experienced health problems suffered from wound infections, especially episiotomy and caesarean section suture line infections (7 per cent) than in Lewisham (5 per cent) or Deptford (3 per cent). Some women in Ashford and Deptford also experienced general discomfort, and perineal discomfort associated with an episiotomy was sometimes reported.

b) Problems experienced by babies

A higher proportion of babies in Deptford (32 per cent) were reported to have experienced health problems between birth and discharge from the midwife than in Lewisham (28 per cent) and Ashford (23 per cent). It is important to note that the figures include babies born with complications identified in pregnancy and premature babies. In addition, some of the babies experienced multiple, often related, health problems of varying severity.

7 per cent of the deliveries in Ashford were pre-term, compared with Lewisham (6 per cent) and 3 per cent in Deptford. Even if some of these were twin births one would not expect the figures for premature babies to change. Of the babies who had experienced problems, over one third in Ashford (35 per cent) and one third in Deptford required special care either immediately after birth or at some stage between birth and discharge from the midwife compared with 27 per cent of the babies in Lewisham.

A higher proportion of babies who had experienced problems in Deptford (12 per cent) were reported to have had feeding problems compared with 8 per cent of the babies with problems in Ashford and Lewisham. In addition, a higher proportion of babies in Deptford had problems with colic or excessive wind (15 per cent), compared with Lewisham (6 per cent) and Ashford (2 per cent). One of the most prevalent problems recorded by midwives was jaundice which was attributed to 38 per cent of the babies with health problems in Lewisham, 32 per cent in Ashford and 21 per cent in Deptford. The data could not confirm the proportion of babies with jaundice that required any intervention such as phototherapy.

14 per cent of babies with problems were reported to have had an infection or pyrexia in Lewisham compared with only 5 per cent in Ashford and 6 per cent in Deptford. In contrast, 14 per cent of babies in Ashford and 9 per cent in Deptford were reported to have had sticky eyes compared to only 3 per cent in Lewisham. Three babies in Lewisham and two in Ashford were reported to have sustained trauma at birth.

It is interesting that both women and babies in Deptford were more likely to have been reported as experiencing health problems compared with either Lewisham or Ashford, although the proportion of women who reported more serious problems was much lower than elsewhere.

What issues were discussed with midwives before discharge?

Giving women the opportunity to discuss problems and issues as they arise requires a flexible approach to the organisation of postnatal visits. We were interested in the issues that midwives discussed during postnatal consultations with women and asked them to record this on the outcome form. We expected that some of the issues would be tailored to the specific needs of each woman, but that the midwives would also focus on other key areas to ensure that women were well-informed, confident and prepared for the early weeks of parenthood.

Individual midwives generally discussed the same issues with women postnatally. For instance, some midwives always recorded having discussed immunisations and the six-weekly postnatal check by the GP, birth registration and family planning. Infant feeding arose in discussions more than any other issue. Women in Deptford were recorded as twice as likely to have discussed this with their midwife (87 per cent) than in Ashford (44 per cent). Discussions about family matters were also given greater emphasis in Deptford, especially in relation to involving partners and siblings and the importance of family support. Maternal care and well-being was discussed with nearly 40 per cent of women in Deptford. However, infant health, immunisations, and general care of a newborn baby were discussed with only a quarter of women in Deptford.

In Lewisham, infant feeding was discussed with two-thirds of the women altogether. More emphasis was placed on infant health, immunisations and the postnatal GP check in Lewisham than elsewhere, although these issues were still discussed with less than half of the women, according to the records. Contraception and family planning were recorded as having been discussed with one third of the Lewisham women, which was more than elsewhere. General care of the newborn was discussed with a quarter of women postnatally and the importance of maternal health and well-being was given the same emphasis. Practical issues such as birth registration was discussed with a quarter of women in Lewisham, a handful in Deptford and appeared not to have been discussed at all in Ashford.

In Ashford, infant feeding was given the most emphasis but still appeared to be discussed with less than half of the women. Health of the infant, immunisations and the six-weekly postnatal check were discussed with over one fifth of women. General maternal health and well-being was also discussed. Contraception and family planning was discussed with over a fifth of women.

In instances where the baby had sustained some trauma or injury at birth midwives always discussed this with women. In all instances where a neonatal death had occurred the focus was primarily on helping and supporting women and their families through the grieving process.

It is clear from the information recorded that some midwives focused on one or two specific areas while others covered a broad range of topics with women. In addition, much depended on the extent to which the midwives recorded the topics they discussed with the women. It is perhaps a matter for concern that there did not appear to be an identifiable programme of issues set out by any of the MGPs which would have enabled a more structured approach to the discussions held with the women. Consultations may be designed to give women an opportunity to discuss their own immediate concerns but this alone may fail to ensure that the information given at the visits is sufficiently comprehensive.

Average age of the baby at discharge from the midwife

Because of the longer period of postnatal care in Deptford (28 days) babies were discharged much later (on average 32 days) than in Lewisham (19 days) or Ashford (14 days) where the MGPs provided postnatal care for 10 days. However, the figures suggest that the midwives in both Ashford and Lewisham did not always discharge babies at exactly 10 days. The average

age of the baby at discharge from the midwife should be seen in relation to the number of postnatal consultations that women received in the three areas from MGP midwives and other professionals.

It is important to note that, although Ashford women were discharged from MGP care on average 18 days before women in Deptford, the number of combined postnatal consultations received by Ashford women was 8.5 compared to 9.1 in Deptford which meant that, in real terms, women still received the same amount of direct postnatal care. It is difficult to tell the extent to which having a known person to contact up to one month after discharge was valued by women in Deptford.

Feeding method at discharge from the midwife

Table 4.10 shows the feeding method at discharge from the midwife. It is important to see this in relation to the average age of the baby at discharge from the MGP. Breast feeding was very successful in all areas but especially in Deptford. 84 per cent of Deptford women were breast feeding at discharge from MGP care, 4 per cent were both breast and bottle feeding and another 2 per cent had breast fed for between 6–10 days before starting to bottle feed.

Table 4.10   Feeding methods at discharge from the MGP midwife

column percentages

	Lewisham	Ashford	Deptford
Breast	50	54	84
Breast and bottle	11	4	4
Breast 1–5 days then bottle	0	1	0
Breast 6–10 days then bottle	0	*	2
Bottle feeding expressed milk	1	1	0
Bottle	35	38	8
Artificial feeding – tube/ intravenous infusion	1	0	0
None – baby died	*	1	2
n.a.	1	2	0
Base: all maternities excluding stillbirths	*(314)*	*(287)*	*(102)*

Half the women in Lewisham and over half in Ashford (54 per cent) were breast feeding at discharge from the midwife, another 11 per cent were both breast and bottle feeding in Lewisham and 4 per cent in Ashford. 1 per cent of women were feeding expressed breast milk in Lewisham and

Ashford, and 1 per cent of women in Ashford were bottle feeding but had breast fed for 5 days or less after birth.

The high breast feeding rates resulted in over one third of women in Lewisham (35 per cent) and Ashford (38 per cent) bottle feeding at discharge from the midwife and only 8 per cent in Deptford.

Continuity of intrapartum care for all deliveries during the monitoring period

One of the objectives of *Changing Childbirth* was that 75 per cent of women should be attended in labour by someone known to them. The MGPs were set up to deliver 200-240 women per annum with a view to attending all of these women in labour and at delivery. We have already seen that none of the MGPs operated at the planned capacity set out in their proposals to SETRHA, albeit for somewhat different reasons. Lewisham and Ashford had a mean monthly booking rate that was higher than their original targets, while, in contrast, Deptford's booking rate was below target.

In view of this, we considered it important to look at the success rate of the MGPs in providing intrapartum continuity of care against the actual number of deliveries for each MGP. So far in this chapter we have concentrated on intrapartum care for our main study group: those women who booked with the MGPs and delivered within the monitoring period. However, because of the workload and activity implications involved when we look at the whole 18-month period, we completed the picture by examining continuity of intrapartum care for all the deliveries from April 1994 to September 1995 presented in Table 3.5, including those women who had booked with the MGP midwives before April 1994.

Deptford

Table 3.5 showed that the Deptford MGP supplied monitoring information for 164 deliveries over the 18-month monitoring period for women who had booked both before or after 1 April 1994. Looking at all the deliveries we found that 94 per cent of all women were attended by their named or primary midwife or by another MGP midwife. The proportion of named midwife attendances for all deliveries was very high but the MGP did not reach the annual target of 200 deliveries even within the 18-month monitoring period. In view of this it is difficult to assess whether the MGP could achieve the same results if it operated at full capacity.

Lewisham

90 per cent of women delivered by the Lewisham MGP over the 18-month monitoring period were attended at delivery by their named midwife or by another MGP midwife. It is clear that in delivering 454 women (see Table 3.5) over the 18-month monitoring period the MGP not only achieved but exceeded its target of providing intrapartum care for 240 women per annum, and also achieved a very high rate of intrapartum continuity of care. However, if the booking rate remains steady at the level noted in Chapter 3, it is unlikely that this continuity of intrapartum care can be continued. This may have a negative impact on maternal satisfaction and create workload difficulties for midwives who have to care for the extra women.

Given the MGP's demonstration that it can meet its target of providing such a high level of intrapartum continuity of care for 240 deliveries per annum, it appears important that extra staffing to meet the demands made on the group should be investigated. Even if the MGP books 10-15 women per annum who deliver elsewhere it would still have around 20 per cent more deliveries than planned under the staffing arrangements.

Ashford

61 per cent of Ashford women were attended during delivery by their named or another MGP midwife. Again, these figures for intrapartum continuity of care should be viewed against the total number of deliveries over the 18-month monitoring period and the MGP's planned capacity of 200 deliveries per annum. The Ashford MGP submitted outcome details for 510 deliveries for the full 18 months, and on the basis of these figures, it can be seen that the MGP could provide 100 per cent continuity of care for 200 women per annum. However, in order to ensure the maintenance of this rate, it is essential that the Ashford MGP adheres to its protocols about eligibility for MGP care on the basis of risk.

Chapter 5

Women's experience of antenatal care

Our interviews with women covered a wide range of topics relating to their views and experience of antenatal and postnatal care and the birth itself. We explored many of the issues raised in *Changing Childbirth*. We wanted to establish to what extent women had been given the information needed to make informed choices, by whom and at what stages in their pregnancy; how women gained access to the services provided by the midwifery group practices; whether and how women were involved in planning a programme of care for pregnancy and delivery, and their experience of care throughout. Other key issues were the extent to which women sought out particular options, or were recipients of care in a less active or less informed sense. For instance, did women make requests for care options themselves? Did they feel they had choices? And what were their reasons for choosing particular care options? This chapter looks at women's experience of antenatal care and Chapter 6 examines their experience of intrapartum and postnatal care.

Our aim was to carry out 300 interviews with women who booked with the midwifery group practices during the monitoring period between April 1994 and the end of September 1995. We intended to conduct 180 interviews with women during pregnancy and 120 follow-up or second interviews with women around one month after delivery. Women who booked or transferred in the first four sampling periods – April, July, October 1994 and January 1995 – were asked at their first interview if they were willing to have a second interview after delivering their babies. Women who booked or transferred in the final two sampling periods (April and July 1995) were not asked for a follow-up interview because it was assumed that they would not have delivered within the monitoring period.

The sampling and selection methods for the interviews are discussed fully in Appendix E. However, the interviewing process itself was not straightforward for a number of reasons: 14 women who had first interviews (usually around 3 months after booking with the MGPs) did not have a follow-up interview after delivery: 8 of these women moved area, 2 women had sick babies and their midwives advised that a follow-up interview would not be appropriate, and the remainder declined a second interview or did not reply. In addition, 12 women had second interviews after delivery but did not have a preliminary interview during pregnancy. In Deptford especially, this occurred because some women who had already received care elsewhere in their current pregnancy transferred to MGP care late in pregnancy and delivered shortly after being selected for a first interview. In other areas a few women could not be contacted during pregnancy and were close to their expected date of delivery or had already delivered when they did agree to be interviewed. In such instances, a partial first interview and a full second interview were carried out after delivery. The partial first interview asked questions about confirmation of pregnancy, to whom women went first to arrange their care for pregnancy and birth, whether they had attended any antenatal classes and whether they had seen a consultant obstetrician during pregnancy.

Overall, 168 full first interviews, 12 partial first interviews and 117 second interviews were carried out with 180 women (65 in Lewisham, 58 in Ashford and 57 in Deptford). It is important to note that the discussion of the characteristics of all the women interviewed relates to this group of 180 women, 12 of whom did not have a full first interview.

Characteristics of women interviewed
The tables in this chapter should be looked at in conjunction with those relating to the characteristics of the women booking with the midwifery group practices during the monitoring period. The 'monitored group' of women referred to in the discussion below relates to *all* women who booked with the MGPs during the monitoring period from April 1994 to the end of September 1995 (see Chapter 3). It does *not* include those who had booked before April 1994.

Age profile
Table 5.1 shows the age profile of women interviewed and underlines the age differences already noted between Deptford and the other pilot areas for women who booked with the MGPs after April 1994. The average age of women interviewed was higher in Deptford (32.7 years) than in Ashford (27.9 years) or in Lewisham (28.9 years).

Women interviewed in Deptford were far less likely to be under 30 than in the other areas: only one fifth of those interviewed in Deptford compared with over half of those interviewed in Lewisham (54 per cent) and Ashford (57 per cent). In fact, 23 per cent in Lewisham and 20 per cent in Ashford were under 25 compared with only 4 per cent in Deptford. One third of women interviewed in Lewisham and Ashford were aged 25–29 years compared with only 16 per cent of women in Deptford.

Table 5.1   Age of all women interviewed

column percentages

	Lewisham	Ashford	Deptford
16–19	3	2	2
20–24	17	21	2
25–29	34	33	16
30–34	37	36	47
35–39	9	7	28
40 plus	0	0	0
n.a.	0	2	0
Mean age	28.9	27.9	32.7
Base: all women interviewed	*(65)*	*(58)*	*(57)*

As many as 80 per cent of the women interviewed in Deptford were 30 years or over, compared with 43 per cent in Ashford and 46 per cent in Lewisham. This reflected the age profile found in the monitored group of women and the differences we had already found across the MGPs.

Marital status

Differences in marital status between women interviewed and the monitored group can be seen by comparing Table 5.2 and the corresponding table in Chapter 3. 78 per cent of the women interviewed in Ashford and 60 per cent in Lewisham were married (compared with 69 per cent of the monitored group of women in Ashford and 53 per cent in Lewisham). In Deptford we found that 49 per cent of those interviewed and in the monitored group were married. Around one sixth of the women interviewed in Lewisham and Deptford were single, compared with 7 per cent of women in Ashford. In Deptford, 32 per cent of those interviewed were living as married, in Ashford 12 per cent and in Lewisham 20 per cent. The remainder of women interviewed in all areas were either divorced or separated.

Table 5.2   Marital status of all women interviewed

column percentages

	Lewisham	Ashford	Deptford
Single	15	7	16
Married	60	78	49
Living as married	20	12	32
Divorced	3	3	4
Separated	2	0	0
Base: all women interviewed	*(65)*	*(58)*	*(57)*

Social class and occupation

a) Women's occupation

Table 5.3 shows that women interviewed in Deptford were three times more likely to be in professional and managerial occupations (56 per cent) than women in Lewisham (17 per cent), compared with one third of the women interviewed in Ashford. This showed a slightly different pattern from that found among the monitored group of women in Lewisham (23 per cent), Ashford (19 per cent) and Deptford (47 per cent).

Table 5.3   Social class/occupation of all women interviewed and their partners

column percentages

| | Women | | | Partners | | |
	Lew	Ash	Dept	Lew	Ash	Dept
Professional I	0	7	2	3	14	11
Intermediate II	17	26	54	11	24	47
Skilled non-manual III N	34	14	5	12	5	11
Skilled manual III M	2	5	2	40	29	7
Semi-skilled IV	3	3	0	6	10	2
Unskilled V	2	0	0	2	5	0
Student	0	3	4	5	3	2
Keeping house/Mother	35	41	19	0	0	0
Unemployed	8	0	14	15	5	12
n.a.	0	0	0	6	4	9
Base: all women interviewed	*(65)*	*(58)*	*(57)*	*(65)*	*(58)*	*(57)*

A higher proportion of women interviewed in Lewisham were in skilled non-manual occupations (34 per cent) than we found in the monitored group (27 per cent). In Ashford comparable figures were 14 per cent among those interviewed and 22 per cent in the monitored group, and in Deptford 5 per cent of those interviewed and 8 per cent in the monitored group. A small proportion of women in all areas were in semi-skilled occupations.

A similar proportion of women interviewed were students in Ashford and Deptford while none of the women interviewed in Lewisham were students. Women in Ashford were twice as likely to be housewives or mothers (41 per cent) than in Deptford (19 per cent): a similar pattern to that found in the monitored group. Over a third of women interviewed in Lewisham were housewives or mothers compared with over a quarter in the monitored group.

While none of the women interviewed in Ashford reported being unemployed, a similar proportion of women interviewed and the monitored group in both Lewisham and Deptford were unemployed. It is important to note again that recording occupations such as unemployed and housewife may differ within and between areas depending on the different interpretation of midwives and the women themselves, so that one woman may say she was a housewife or mother but could be reported by a midwife as unemployed, or the other way round.

b) Partner's occupation

Over half the partners of women interviewed in Deptford were in professional or managerial occupations, which was rather higher than that reported for the monitored group (49 per cent). A higher proportion of partners in Ashford were also in professional and managerial occupations (38 per cent) than in the monitored group (28 per cent). A lower proportion of partners of women interviewed in Lewisham were in professional and managerial occupations (14 per cent) than in the monitored group (24 per cent).

A similar proportion of partners were in skilled non-manual occupations in all areas as found in the monitored group. Around the same proportion of partners in Lewisham and Ashford were in manual occupations for both groups, but 9 per cent of partners in Deptford were in manual occupations compared with 17 per cent of Deptford partners in the monitored group. A slightly higher proportion were unemployed in Lewisham than in the monitored group while more were unemployed in the monitored group in Ashford.

The occupations of partners of women interviewed reflected the pattern found in the monitored group, with partners in Lewisham and Ashford being most commonly in skilled manual occupations, while in contrast, partners in Deptford were most commonly in professional or managerial occupations.

To summarise, the Deptford women and their partners were predominantly in middle-class occupations. Lewisham women were more likely to be in non-manual skilled occupations and both Lewisham and Ashford women were more likely to be housewives or mothers than the Deptford women.

Ethnic group

Table 5.4 indicates more ethnic diversity in Lewisham and Deptford than in Ashford, but despite this the overwhelming majority of women were of white ethnic origin: a similar pattern to that found among the monitored group of women.

Table 5.4   Ethnic group of all women interviewed

column percentages

	Lewisham	Ashford	Deptford
White	82	97	79
Black Caribbean	12	0	7
Black African	5	2	5
Black British	0	0	2
Indian	0	2	2
Pakistani	0	0	0
Bangladeshi	0	0	0
Chinese	0	0	0
Vietnamese	0	0	5
Mixed race	2	0	0
Base: all women interviewed	*(65)*	*(58)*	*(57)*

82 per cent of women interviewed in Lewisham were of white ethnic origin, 19 per cent of women were from non-white ethnic minority groups and 17 per cent were from Black minority groups alone. This was similar to the monitored group.

97 per cent of the women interviewed in Ashford were of white ethnic origin which was similar to the monitored group. The remainder of women were Black African or Indian.

In Deptford a slightly higher proportion of women interviewed were of white ethnic origin (79 per cent) than in the monitored group (73 per cent). 21 per cent of women were from non-white ethnic minority groups and 14 per cent of women were from Black ethnic minority groups alone.

Housing status

The living circumstances of women interviewed and the monitored group were similar across the different areas. Table 5.5 shows that the proportion of owner occupation in Lewisham and Ashford for women who were interviewed and the monitored group was similar: 48 per cent of women interviewed in Lewisham and 59 per cent in Ashford were owner-occupiers. 68 per cent of the women interviewed in Deptford were owner-occupiers compared with 55 per cent of the monitored group.

Nearly the same proportion of the monitored group and women interviewed in Ashford were private tenants, while a lower proportion of women interviewed in Lewisham and Deptford were private tenants. Council tenancy was more common among women interviewed in Lewisham than in the monitored group and less common among women interviewed in Ashford. A similar proportion of the monitored group and women interviewed in Deptford were council tenants. The remainder of women in all areas were living with relatives. Other women lived in housing association accommodation or at temporary addresses.

Table 5.5   Housing status of all women interviewed

column percentages

	Lewisham	Ashford	Deptford
Owner-occupier	48	59	68
Private tenant	3	15	7
Council tenant	38	14	18
Hotel or hostel	2	0	0
Living with relatives	5	7	2
Housing Association	5	2	4
Temporary address	0	2	2
Other living arrangements	0	2	0
Base: all women interviewed	*(65)*	*(58)*	*(57)*

Number of previous pregnancies

Table 5.6 shows a similar pattern between the monitored group of women and the women interviewed in Ashford and Deptford in relation to previous pregnancies. Overall, 82 per cent of women interviewed in Deptford and 72 per cent in Ashford had had previous pregnancies, compared with 79 per cent of women in Deptford and 70 per cent in Ashford in the monitored group. 78 per cent of women interviewed in Lewisham had had previous pregnancies compared with 69 per cent of the monitored group.

Table 5.6   Previous pregnancies of all women interviewed

column percentages

	Lewisham	Ashford	Deptford
None	22	28	18
1	31	41	33
2	20	16	21
3 plus	27	15	28
Base: all women interviewed	*(65)*	*(58)*	*(57)*

Number of children

Table 5.7 shows that over two-thirds of women interviewed in all areas had had one or more children before the current pregnancy. Nearly half the women in Deptford had one child, compared with 45 per cent in Ashford and 32 per cent in Lewisham. A higher proportion of women in Lewisham had 2 children (23 per cent) than in Ashford (14 per cent) or Deptford (11 per cent). Rather surprisingly, 12 per cent of women in Lewisham and 9 per cent in Ashford and Deptford had 3 or more children which is higher than the national figures. It can be seen that a relatively high number of the women interviewed could compare their current maternity care with previous care.

Table 5.7   Number of children of all women interviewed

column percentages

	Lewisham	Ashford	Deptford
None	32	33	32
1	32	45	29
2	23	14	11
3 plus	12	9	9
Base: all women interviewed	(65)	(58)	(57)

When did women have their first interview?

168 women had a full first interview (62 in Lewisham, 55 in Ashford and 51 in Deptford) which looked at a broad range of issues relating to their antenatal care. It is important to note that the following discussion relates to the antenatal care the women had had before their first interview and therefore does not cover the whole antenatal period. The average number of weeks gestation of women at the first interview was 25.8 weeks in Lewisham, 23.7 in Ashford and 29 in Deptford.

Access to the service

We asked women how they confirmed pregnancy and to whom they went first to arrange their care. The two main routes to arranging care were via the GP practice or by a direct approach to the midwives or the MGP. Women in all areas were more likely to arrange care through their GP but the proportion varied considerably across the three areas.

Over three-quarters of women in Lewisham and Deptford confirmed their pregnancy through a home test or pharmacy test, compared with 71 per cent of women in Ashford. 20 per cent of women in Ashford, 17 per cent in Lewisham but only 8 per cent in Deptford had a test at their GP practice. Some women went to a family planning clinic or had a test carried out through their MGP midwife, and a few women confirmed pregnancy while having investigations for infertility.

Having confirmed pregnancy, 98 per cent of women in Lewisham went to a GP first to arrange their care, while the remainder went to a practice nurse or midwife at the GP practice. In Ashford, 73 per cent went to their GP first, most of the rest went to the MGP, while one woman went directly to the hospital to arrange for a particular hospital midwife to care for her. In Deptford, 57 per cent of women went to a GP first and the remainder went directly to the MGP. Women in Deptford were least likely to go to their GP to arrange care first which is possibly due to the fact that a relatively high proportion of Deptford women had received care from particular MGP midwives in previous pregnancies.

In Lewisham and Ashford it was assumed that women would go to their GP first and then be referred to the MGP, although it was also envisaged that some women would go to the MGP directly. In Deptford direct access was facilitated by the walk-in shopfront, but women could also be referred by professionals such as GPs or community midwives. However, a high proportion of self referrals were women already known to the MGP midwives.

Women who went to their GP first to arrange their care

The question of actively choosing a GP as the first point of contact did not arise for many women, since many were not aware that they could go elsewhere to discuss and arrange their care. Women went to their GP as a formality or because they thought that was the normal route, but this was more often reported by women in Lewisham (77 per cent) than in Deptford (59 per cent) or Ashford (55 per cent). Other women went to the GP first because they had done so for previous pregnancies (Lewisham 6 per cent, Ashford 15 per cent and Deptford 10 per cent). One woman in Lewisham explained: 'On the box (home test kit) it says go to the doctor as soon as you know you're pregnant.' Another woman in Ashford said: 'You always go to your doctor. You never think of going anywhere else.'

Nearly a quarter of the women in Ashford (23 per cent), and 10 per cent in Lewisham and Deptford went to their GPs to get further confirmation of pregnancy. Others went for reasons such as problems experienced in early pregnancy, or worries about the recurrence of problems experienced in previous pregnancies, or because they had had shared care involving their GP before.

What information did women receive about the MGPs from their GP?

Because MGP midwives in Lewisham and Ashford were based in 'host' GP practices we expected those GPs to give information to women about the MGPs. Instead there appeared to be a rather haphazard approach to information-giving at this stage. Women in Lewisham were more likely to receive information from their GP about the MGP (61 per cent) than women in Ashford (45 per cent) or Deptford (17 per cent). The number of women in Ashford who said that they did not receive information about the MGPs from their GPs is remarkably high, considering that these GP practices were chosen to take part in the evaluation.

If GPs did give information to women, they often mentioned that the MGP was a new scheme where care was provided by a midwife, with a general explanation of what the new system of care offered, referring in some instances to specific details such as the possibility of home visits and continuity of antenatal care. One Ashford woman said: 'He explained the system has changed and there's a group of midwives who are quite capable of taking care of me and I'd be assigned my own midwife.'

Could women who went to their GP first choose care options?

It became apparent that there was no consistent approach to presenting care options to women by GPs within or across the pilot sites. Although most women went to their GP first to discuss and arrange their care in Lewisham and Ashford, it was envisaged that MGP midwives would present options to women during the booking appointment. However, by the time women met an MGP midwife, some said that they had already been informed by their GP that they would be cared for by the MGP. Our interviews with women indicated that, despite going to the GP practice to discuss care arrangements, some women, particularly in Ashford, had very little discussion with their GP and were either advised to make an appointment with the MGP or had an appointment made for them.

Only around half of the women who went to their GP first in Lewisham, 30 per cent in Ashford and 28 per cent in Deptford, reported that they were offered a choice by their GP of who would be in charge of their care during their pregnancy and for the birth of their baby. 39 per cent of women in Lewisham said that they were *not* offered a choice of care options by their GP, compared with 30 per cent in Ashford and 48 per cent in Deptford. A further 8 per cent of women in Lewisham and Ashford and 21 per cent in Deptford indicated that they were not offered a choice because they requested a specific care option. The remainder of women in all areas noted that the midwife rather than the GP had offered a choice of care options (3 per cent in Lewisham and Deptford and 33 per cent of women in Ashford).

If women were not offered a choice by their GP what were they told about their care arrangements?

Of the 25 women who were not offered a choice in Lewisham, 14 were told by their GP that they would receive MGP care, 7 were not told anything specific about their care, 3 were told that they would have shared care and one could not remember.

In Ashford, 22 of the 24 women not offered a choice were either told that they would receive MGP care or were not told anything specific about their care. One was told that she would have shared care involving the hospital and one woman could not remember.

In Deptford 9 of the 15 women were told that they would have some form of shared care, 3 were referred to the antenatal clinic at the hospital, 2 said that they were told nothing and another said that her GP referred her to the MGP.

It was perhaps surprising that some women said that the GP had not mentioned anything at all about their care. A woman in Ashford said: 'I know a bit because of having a baby before. It wasn't until I had spoken to the midwife that I knew about the arrangement and there was no mention, except from the midwife, about the special GP practices involved.'

The fact that women themselves expected more information and input from their GP was noted by another woman in Ashford who said: 'He did nothing. He said book at three months to see the midwife. I was rather frightened because it was my first pregnancy and I expected him to do more.'

The high proportion of women who felt that they were not offered a choice of care options by their GP could be related to the fact that there did not appear to be a clear protocol in any area for dealing with women who went to their GP to discuss care arrangements. In Ashford for instance, some women who went to their GP practice had a confirmation of pregnancy test and were referred directly to the MGP by the GP receptionist. (This group of women are referred to later under women who went directly to the MGP.) Other women had a brief discussion with their GP before being advised to book with the MGP midwife.

The variety of experiences reported by women who went to their GP to discuss care seemed to result from the individual interpretations of the GPs themselves about their role in guiding and advising women at this stage. It seems likely that the confusion felt by some of the women we interviewed in Lewisham and Ashford (where MGP midwives were based in 'host practices') could have been easily avoided if women had been informed that they would have a preliminary discussion about care options with their GP, but that this would be followed by a more detailed discussion with the MGP midwife at their first consultation or booking visit.

For women who said they were offered a choice by their GP about who would look after them in pregnancy and for the birth of their baby, the most common option offered by GPs in Lewisham and Ashford was MGP care, while in Deptford it was GP care itself.

What care options did women choose and why?

If women were offered a choice, most chose midwifery care rather than any other care option: 26 of the 31 women offered a choice in Lewisham, 9 of the 12 women in Ashford, and 4 of the 8 women in Deptford chose MGP care. Most of the rest opted for some form of shared care arrangement and one Ashford woman opted for consultant care. Half of the women who went to their GP in Lewisham and Ashford were told that even if they chose a midwife to care for them they could still see a GP or a consultant obstetrician, while around 20 per cent of women in Deptford were told this.

Women who opted for midwifery care mainly said that they wanted continuity of care, some women liked what their GP had said about the care, while others wanted specific features such as home visits or the opportunity to have a home birth. A preference for the professional expertise of midwives was reflected in the comments made by a woman in Ashford: 'I believe in the midwife being the most qualified to help with childbirth. It is not an illness. It doesn't need intervention from a doctor, and I want continuity of care.' A woman in Deptford said: 'All the way along I knew I wanted a midwife I knew and who knew me, and it wasn't part of a lottery where you get whatever's available at the hospital.'

In Deptford the women who opted for shared care said that they wanted a home birth but still wanted GP care. One said: 'I was interested in having a home birth. My GP didn't have an obstetric service but I liked my GP so I opted for shared care because she knows us as a family.' Negative experiences of hospital care in the past were also mentioned. Another woman in Deptford explained: 'At my first birth the community midwife was not available and someone else took over. I don't know what happened but we certainly had a personality clash. That was more traumatic than the birth. She kept telling me to hurry on or she would have to induce me.'

Women who went to a midwife first

We have already seen that women in Deptford were much more likely to go directly to the MGP than women in Ashford, while only one woman in Lewisham did so. Nearly three-quarters of the women we interviewed in Deptford who went directly to the MGP knew a particular midwife in the MGP through previous pregnancies. Another fifth were introduced to the MGP by colleagues, friends and relatives with experience of some of the MGP midwives in the past. A few women in Deptford had seen the advertisement for the service on the shopfront.

One woman in Deptford told us how she had met her midwife: 'She was my NCT teacher during my last pregnancy. I had severe postnatal depression and she was very supportive. I'd had my first baby in hospital so I rang her as soon as I found out I was pregnant and asked if she would look after me this time.'

Over half the women in Ashford who went directly to the MGP already knew or had heard of a particular midwife through relatives, friends or colleagues. The remainder of the women were told by the receptionist at their GP practice to contact the MGP directly following confirmation of their pregnancy test. These women went via the GP practice rather than directly to the MGP, but had not had any discussion about their care with their GP. The women who went directly to a midwife in Ashford were either offered a choice about who would care for them (12 women) or sought particular options (3 women).

Over three-quarters of the women who went directly to a midwife in Deptford (17 women) said that they had a specific care option in mind. Three said they were offered a choice of care options but two said that they had not been offered a choice at all. For the women who were offered a choice, the most frequent options were MGP care, followed by GP care and hospital care. All but one of the women offered a choice opted for MGP care.

How were appointments made with the MGP?

The approach to setting up MGP appointments differed across the pilot sites, with midwives in Lewisham mostly contacting the women themselves. One woman in Lewisham told us: 'I wasn't particularly impressed with the doctor. I phoned the surgery again and asked to see another doctor who explained everything to me and gave me a choice of hospitals or the DOMINO scheme. The practice wrote to me and said my care would be at Lewisham. (The midwife) rang me and said she was going to be my midwife and made a booking appointment.'

In Ashford a small proportion of women said that they set up the appointment themselves, but for most women the appointment was made via the GP practice by a practice nurse, receptionist or the GP.

In Deptford, women usually telephoned or called into the MGP office. One woman in Deptford told us how she contacted the MGP initially: 'I called in when I think I was 12 weeks pregnant and asked them what they were about and decided I'd like to be with them. There are certain categories like having income support or having manic depression, which made me all right to be a client.'

Choosing place of birth – options and decisions

The opportunity for women to choose a place of birth and being able to alter that decision was emphasised in *Changing Childbirth*. In our discussions with women it became clear that a high proportion of women in all areas (92 per cent in Ashford, 86 per cent in Lewisham and 81 per cent in Deptford) had decided where they wanted to give birth at the first consultation or booking visit with their midwife. However, there were clear differences even at this stage in women's preferences for place of birth across the three areas.

59 per cent of the women in Deptford wanted a home birth, compared with 18 per cent of women in Lewisham and as few as 5 per cent in Ashford. In contrast, 87 per cent of Ashford women had planned to have a hospital birth, compared with 68 per cent in Lewisham and 22 per cent in Deptford. The remainder of women in all areas were undecided. A similar pattern could be seen in Ashford and Deptford for the monitored group of women although a higher proportion of the women interviewed in Lewisham were undecided about place of birth.

One of the main messages to emerge from our interviews with women was that they were certainly not a homogeneous group. The interplay of personal, family, social and organisational factors produced an interesting diversity which highlights the challenge in developing and tailoring services to meet women's needs. Even if women expressed similar preferences for place of birth, their reasons for doing so were not necessarily the same. In addition, women who were cared for by the same MGP had somewhat different experiences of past care and different expectations for their current pregnancy, which shaped their decisions on where they wanted to deliver their baby.

Why did women make the choices they did?

Some women who chose a home birth in Lewisham felt that it would be more relaxing and comfortable at home than in hospital. As one woman in Lewisham put it: 'When you're in your own home you feel a little more in control and relaxed and I don't want to spend the whole of my labour yelling and screaming at people to leave me alone, strapping me to monitors - and that won't be good for the progress of my labour.'

Previous negative experiences of hospital care influenced other women as a woman in Lewisham explained: 'It's my third pregnancy and I wanted to be at home. The after care at (the hospital) was non-existent. They didn't show you how to bath your baby or even feed it.' A woman in Deptford said: 'I haven't had pleasant experiences with hospitals, but I was anxious about a home birth and wanted to find out more.' Other women chose to have a home birth in order to avoid hospital technology or because of a previous good experience of a home birth.

For other women necessity rather than choice seemed to influence deci-sions and some felt that a home birth was not a realistic option because of their circumstances. For instance, the home environment or physical sur-roundings rather than the perceived danger of giving birth at home con-cerned some women. A Deptford woman explained: 'Because of my last experience at the hospital I know I would have been more comfortable at home but I couldn't be at home in our first place – it was a flat with very thin walls.' A woman in Lewisham who opted for a hospital birth said: 'I live in a one bedroom flat and the walls are like paper. I'd be better off in hospital.' Other women had other concerns about home births as a woman in Ashford explained: 'Mainly because my partner would be very against a home delivery, I didn't even consider it.'

The most common reason given by women who wanted a hospital birth, especially in Ashford, was because it felt safer. This view was reflected by a woman in Lewisham: 'If anything goes wrong the equipment's there. I couldn't bear it at home – let the professionals take over.' An Ashford woman said: 'I didn't want to have it at home, just in case I have a prob-lem with my asthma. And I didn't want blood on my cream carpet!'

Practical concerns about giving birth at home were mentioned by others such as this woman in Ashford: 'I don't want to make a mess on the carpet – we're just in the middle of redecorating! I'd prefer to go to the hospital, because if I need anything, it'll be there and I shan't have to rush across Ashford.'

Some women felt that they would be better off in hospital because of complications with previous labours, while others, especially in their first pregnancy, felt that hospital would be safer for them. A few women favoured the extra pain relief options available in hospital and the oppor-tunity to rest and be cared for by professional staff. A woman in Ashford who wanted a waterbirth in hospital said: 'To be honest, you get more rest at hospital. When I had my daughter, I wasn't even in six hours and I had such problems afterwards.'

Were women offered a choice of place of birth?

We asked women if they felt they had been offered a choice about place of birth by their midwife. 85 per cent of women in Lewisham felt they had been offered a choice compared with 78 per cent in Deptford and 73 per cent in Ashford. A further 8 per cent of women in Lewisham and Deptford and 11 per cent in Ashford indicated that they were not offered a choice of place of birth because they had requested a particular option. In all areas the most frequently cited option was a home birth, followed by hospital birth. Specific hospitals were emphasised by all three MGPs, usually in their own local area.

While a large proportion of women felt they were offered a choice, many women noted that some options were given more or less emphasis by midwives, depending on their own views and preferences. A woman in Ashford said: 'I know she's quite keen on a waterbirth and she'd like me to have it at home, but I still haven't decided yet.' A Lewisham woman said of her midwife: 'She explained that the group practice were quite keen on home births even for a first baby, but she said that it's entirely up to me and I can change my mind at any time.' A Deptford woman said that her midwife had a definite preference for home birth but that the choice was still hers: 'She's going along with what I want to do. Initially I was worried that she might be evangelical about a home birth, but she's assured me that if I feel I need to go into hospital, there is no problem.'

It became clear that some women felt that it might be difficult to exercise choice in the face of the emphasis, either intentional or unintentional, that midwives tended to place on their own preferred options. Many different examples were given by women where they reported that the emphasis on a care option given by the midwife was not one that they themselves had favoured, resulting in women feeling unsure about whether they had made the right choice. A woman in Deptford explained how she felt that although she had opted for a hospital birth, the emphasis at the antenatal classes was on home births and said: 'I have noticed that it's more geared towards home births. I sort of feel that maybe I should be having it at home.'

Keeping options open and changing preferences for place of birth

Keeping options open was important for some women. A woman in Lewisham noted: 'I'm waiting to see how things go. If there are any problems I'll go into hospital. Otherwise I'll have a home birth.' A Deptford woman said: 'I'd like to stay at home as long as possible, and if possible, have a home birth. But I'm not being dogmatic about it because you never know what is going to happen.'

When we spoke to women about their preference for place of birth at the time of the interview, some had changed their minds from their initial preference and some had made up their minds. Four women had changed their preference from home to hospital (2 in Lewisham, 1 in Ashford and 1 in Deptford). A Lewisham woman told us why she had changed her mind: 'Just in case there are any complications. And it was my agreement with my husband who wanted me to have a little bit of rest before coming home. The baby is breech and hasn't turned yet – it's just me worrying I suppose. That's what changed my mind.' 5 women in Lewisham and 1 in Deptford opted for a hospital birth after a period of indecision and 7 women opted for a home birth (2 in Lewisham, 1 in Ashford and 4 in Deptford).

By the time of the first interview, two-thirds of women in Deptford planned to have a home birth, compared with 16 per cent in Lewisham and only 6 per cent in Ashford. 87 per cent of women planned to have a hospital birth in Ashford, 77 per cent in Lewisham and only 24 per cent in Deptford. The remainder of women in all areas were still undecided at the time of the first interview.

Continuity of care

Having the support of trusted and familiar professionals is one of the key aspects of woman-centred care. We therefore asked women in their first interview how much it actually mattered that they had the same midwife both for their antenatal care and at the birth of their baby. Women in Deptford felt more strongly about having the same midwife throughout – 86 per cent said that this mattered a lot to them compared with over three-quarters of the Lewisham women and over two-thirds in Ashford.

22 per cent of women in Ashford indicated that continuity mattered to some extent, compared with 15 per cent in Lewisham and 8 per cent in Deptford. A relatively small proportion of women in all areas said that continuity did not matter at all – 10 per cent in Lewisham, 9 per cent in Ashford and 6 per cent in Deptford.

Women's experience of their care during pregnancy seemed to shape their views on the value or otherwise of intrapartum continuity of care. An Ashford woman said: 'Now I've seen her and know her, I'd be gutted it she wasn't there. I feel I have been spoilt, my friend kept seeing different people when she was pregnant.' A woman in Lewisham noted: 'I don't think I'll be focused when the time comes, as long as the baby comes out! It would be nice if she was there, because it would be nice to know the person telling you what to do.' Another Lewisham woman said of her antenatal care: 'It's really nice, she makes you feel you are a person, not just a piece of meat. It's worked out really well. When I was working she came to see me on Saturdays so I didn't have to take time off work.'

A woman in Ashford recognised the value of continuity of care but was doubtful of being attended by her midwife in labour and said: 'It's important to me, but from what I hear, they hardly ever manage to be there at the birth.' Other women distinguished between antenatal and intrapartum continuity of care and expressed different views in relation to both. An Ashford woman said: 'I like the same person going through, but when I'm in labour I don't care.' Another Ashford woman said: 'For the first pregnancy I wanted X and was disappointed when I didn't get her. But this time I don't really care. When it comes to it, you don't care.'

Antenatal and intrapartum continuity of care

Nearly three-quarters of women in Deptford said that they had been seen by other midwives antenatally, probably because women in Deptford were cared for by two midwives. Nearly all of these had seen another MGP midwife, and two-thirds of the women said that they had seen only one other midwife. 20 per cent of women (11) in Ashford reported seeing other midwives. Of these, 8 had seen an MGP midwife, 2 a hospital midwife and 1 an MGP and hospital midwife. Two-thirds of the women had seen only one other midwife and the remainder had seen several. 23 per cent of women (14) in Lewisham had seen other midwives. All said that this was an MGP midwife and all but one had seen only one other midwife.

Not surprisingly, women's views about being seen by other midwives or other professionals were often influenced by what happened at their consultations and how they thought they were treated. In Lewisham for instance, one woman said: 'You get used to knowing one person – going to the hospital is a load of rubbish. You just see junior doctors in little side wards. You never see a midwife.' A woman in Ashford said of the hospital staff: 'They never explained anything. They walked in and took your temperature and that was it.'

The majority of women in all areas said that they did not mind seeing other midwives. Disappointment was expressed by only one woman in Deptford, two in Lewisham and three in Ashford who had seen other midwives.

Generally women said they did not mind seeing other MGP midwives because they welcomed different opinions, because the midwives had similar ways of working or because it just did not matter. A Deptford woman was not concerned at all: '...because both midwives were involved at the initial booking session. I actually find the idea of a pair of midwives caring for me reassuring. If it were just one I would be anxious about what would happen if she were called away.' Another woman in Deptford recognised that there could never be certainty about continuity of care and noted that: 'In an ideal world you would have one person the whole time but there's no absolute guarantee that she'll be around for the birth, so it's practical to get to know someone else.'

Planning antenatal care

Had women been asked whether they wanted anyone else such as a partner to be involved in planning their care? Women in Deptford were twice as likely to have been asked this (80 per cent) than women in Ashford (36 per cent). 56 per cent of the women we spoke to in Lewisham said that they were asked. Some of the women said that it was implicit that partners would be involved.

Women clearly valued having partners and children involved at their consultations and scans rather than being treated as peripheral or unimportant. A woman in Ashford explained that her midwife first determined whether the pregnancy was planned before moving on to the issue of involving others in planning care. She explained how her partner was left out completely during a scan at the hospital: 'We had such a disappointing time at the scan. (My partner) was completely ignored, just left holding the coats.' A Lewisham woman told us how her children were included by the MGP midwife in her antenatal consultations: 'The children have always been here and she makes them part of it. She lets them listen to the heartbeat and blow up the blood pressure pump. She's brilliant with them. My partner's always at work. We do talk about him though.'

Appointments built around the availability of partners were valued. A woman in Lewisham noted that because of the opportunity to have evening visits, her husband could be there: 'My husband gets involved in those consultations. I don't have to tell him what (the midwife) says second hand.'

Where did antenatal consultations take place and did women have a choice about where they would be seen?

Women in Ashford were less likely to have been offered a choice (62 per cent) about where they would be seen than women in Lewisham (87 per cent) or in Deptford (82 per cent). In Lewisham and Deptford the most common option offered to women were home visits, while in Ashford the most common option offered to women were GP practice-based visits.

20 per cent of the women in Lewisham reported that they could choose a venue which was most convenient to them compared with 17 per cent of women in Deptford and 9 per cent in Ashford. A few women reported that they requested particular options themselves, while others reported that they were told where their consultations would be or that the midwife knew them well enough to decide what suited them best. A Deptford woman described how her midwife arranged the place and time of her consultations: 'She asked when and where should they be. I said at the weekend, not expecting her to say yes. It's been really nice, she comes at the weekends when (my partner) is here. She'll come on Sundays or Saturdays.' A woman in Lewisham explained why she opted for home visits: 'I chose here because of convenience. More than that, it makes pregnancy less punctuated with hospital/surgery visits. Less waiting time for appointments, less time off work. It made it a normal part of my day.'

84 per cent of women in Lewisham reported having mostly home visits and the remainder mentioned GP surgery visits. One woman in Lewisham and 2 in Ashford said that they had mostly hospital consultations. Only 18 per cent of women reported having home visits in Ashford with the remainder having mostly GP surgery visits, while in Deptford 90 per cent of women said that they had mostly home visits, others had visits at the MGP office and a few women mentioned other venues. This reinforces the findings from the forms completed by the midwives on the location of consultations during the 18-month monitoring period, where we found that the majority of consultations in Deptford and Lewisham were home-

based while GP practice-based consultations were most common in Ashford (see Chapter 3).

Working with other professionals

Working in partnership in the best interests of women has been highlighted as one of the key objectives in *Changing Childbirth* and this was discussed during interviews with midwives, GPs and consultant obstetricians. However, we were interested in women's views of how the professionals involved in their care had worked together and asked women if they felt that there had been effective team work.

A quarter of the women interviewed in Deptford and nearly one fifth of those in Lewisham felt that the professionals involved in their care did not work effectively as a team, compared with only 9 per cent of women in Ashford. Women in Ashford were more likely to report that there was effective team work (71 per cent) than women in Lewisham (52 per cent) or in Deptford (41 per cent).

In many instances women highlighted what amounted to different ways of working which perhaps are not unique to the midwifery group practices and indeed are likely to reflect different philosophies of care and approaches to service provision between different professional groups, and even within professional groups across different settings. As recipients of care, women were extremely well placed to make judgements about their care. However, some of the observations should be treated with caution because they often relate to specific events and professional treatment which the women found unacceptable.

Nonetheless, it is clear from women's comments that their experience of care was shaped by a whole spectrum of people and events and that transforming the face of maternity care must be an inter-disciplinary effort in order to achieve a seamless service. While consultant obstetricians, GPs and midwives are important players, women's experiences of care can go beyond clinics and consultation rooms to include other hospital departments, other hospital doctors and reception or ancillary staff. The improvements envisaged in *Changing Childbirth* require some far-reaching changes across the service in general which means that the focus of change and the investment of effort should not be limited to a few professional groups.

In expressing their views on whether professionals worked effectively together, women were very clear about where the difficulties lay and which professionals worked least and most effectively together. One woman commenting on teamwork in Ashford said: 'I think the consultant obstetrician and the midwife more so than the GP. I am always processed by the GP – another one in and another one out. But I don't feel like that with the consultant obstetrician or the midwife.' Another woman in Ashford said of the relationship between her GP and midwife: 'They function very effectively as a team. He takes on her cases while she is on holiday.'

Women's views seemed to be heavily influenced by particular episodes, events or mistakes which arose in their dealings with the hospital. A woman in Ashford said: 'The first time I went into hospital they didn't have my blood results even though I knew (the midwife) had done them, so they had to do another lot. Then the third time I went they said that my blood count was low and I needed to take iron. When I got home I looked at the blood results and saw that they weren't even mine. They don't seem to be communicating, not really.'

A Deptford woman explained how something had arisen during a scan at the hospital which alarmed her: 'The scanographer was not forthcoming with answers or an explanation. They have identified problems and alarmed me but there was no back-up in terms of support or answers. The midwife is trying to get the information for me.'

Other women felt that some professionals were not keen to be involved in their care or that they were reluctant partners in care. A Lewisham woman said: 'I don't think the GP is too bothered. I think she just wants to push all the work on to the midwife and I haven't had any evidence of communication between them.' Another Lewisham woman noted: 'My doctor's absolutely useless. She did so little at my 16 week appointment, so when she suggested I see her again at 20 weeks I said I'd stick with the midwife under this scheme, and she didn't seem to know the scheme, even though she put me on it in the first place.'

Communication was an area which some women felt was problematic. This was possibly caused by the absence of guidelines or communication protocols, which appeared to be a major problem in the setting up of the midwifery group practices (see Chapter 8 for the views of GPs), but also because of a reluctance on the part of professionals to share information and to keep others informed, which is a recognised problem in interprofessional relationships in any case.

This was noted in particular by women in Deptford. One expressed concern because her midwife was not aware of a consultation that had occurred with a consultant obstetrician: 'I don't think the midwife was told at all. I think this is the weakest part of the scheme. I think the cooperation is adequate and no more. Probably with a pilot a lot more GPs and hospital people don't know what's going on. It's a slight annoyance for them (the midwives) because they don't fit into the system. They are not established as an option.'

Another Deptford woman mentioned the lack of communication between her midwife and GP and said: 'At no point is there any mention of liaison. When she (the midwife) took my blood tests she didn't pass them on to my knowledge. It's very separate. I find it a problem actually. I don't know who to ask questions of. I think it's up to me to liaise between the two.'

In other instances women had clearly decided to by-pass their GP and one woman in Deptford said: 'I haven't even told my GP I'm pregnant.' There were many other examples cited by women of underlying and sometimes overt displays of tension in professional relations. A woman in Ashford explained what happened when she went to see her GP for an antenatal appointment: 'When I went for my medical, he said, "What do I do? With this scheme I don't know where I stand."'

A Deptford woman said – 'I get the feeling that there is competition for being in charge and in control' – while another Deptford woman said – 'The midwife had a lot of trouble getting the results of my blood tests from the GP. I think the midwifery practice are ready to work with the GP but she's not keen on working with them.'

The feeling of being 'caught in the middle' and the pressure of having to choose one professional at the expense of another was noted by a woman in Lewisham who identified what she liked least about the service: 'Only that you choose between the doctor and the midwife. It seems like a battle, having to choose.'

Were women offered a choice of seeing a consultant obstetrician?

Changing Childbirth emphasises the role of consultant obstetricians as the lead professionals for women with complicated pregnancies, but it also points to the need for women with uncomplicated pregnancies to be offered the opportunity to meet an obstetrician during pregnancy.

We asked women if they had been given the opportunity to see a consultant obstetrician. Over half of the women interviewed in Ashford (58 per cent) said that they had, compared with 40 per cent of women in Lewisham and 29 per cent in Deptford. It is important to bear in mind that these figures relate to what had happened up to the time when women were interviewed and that more women could have been offered a choice at a later stage in pregnancy. We have already seen that the average number of weeks gestation of women at their first interview in Lewisham was 25.8 weeks, 23.7 weeks in Ashford and 29 weeks in Deptford.

Although women in Deptford were less likely to have had the option of seeing a consultant obstetrician than women elsewhere, a higher proportion of women in Deptford reported that they had actually seen a consultant or another hospital doctor (33 per cent) than in Ashford (25 per cent) or Lewisham (21 per cent). Most of the referrals in all areas were made because of problems or complications experienced by women in their current or in previous pregnancies. Only 2 of the 14 women who saw a consultant or other hospital doctor in Ashford, and 2 of the 17 women in Deptford requested a referral themselves. None of the 13 women in Lewisham had requested the referral.

The vast majority of the women who were referred to a consultant or other hospital doctor in all areas felt that the reason for the referral had been explained clearly to them. None of the women were accompanied by an MGP midwife to the consultations in Ashford and only 2 were accompanied by their midwife in Lewisham. In contrast, 7 of the 17 women were accompanied by their midwife to these consultations in Deptford, reinforcing the finding in Chapters 2 and 3 that midwives in Deptford accompanied women on specialist appointments more often than elsewhere.

Communication between midwives and the women

Over and over again women mentioned the difficulties they had experienced in the past in discussing concerns and queries about their care and in having their views and wishes taken into account. The MGPs were very successful in ensuring that women did not have the same negative experiences. All the women in Lewisham and Ashford and all but 2 women in Deptford felt they could talk freely with their midwife. All the women in Lewisham and all but one in Ashford and Deptford felt that their midwife always explained things clearly. An overwhelming majority of women in Lewisham and all the women in Ashford and Deptford said that their views and wishes were respected by their midwives.

Satisfaction with the MGP service at the first interview

Maternal satisfaction was identified by consultant obstetricians, GPs and midwives as one of the criteria for assessing the success of the MGPs. It is also pivotal to the issue of replicability of the MGP models of care. We asked women during their first interview how satisfied they were with the service they had received from their MGP up to that point. A very high proportion of women in all areas were very satisfied with the service from their MGP. 90 per cent of the women interviewed in Deptford were very satisfied with the service and the remainder were fairly satisfied. In Lewisham 84 per cent of women were very satisfied, 13 per cent were fairly satisfied and only one woman reported being dissatisfied with the service. In Ashford 82 per cent of women were very satisfied, 15 per cent were fairly satisfied and two women were dissatisfied.

The main factor which led to women's satisfaction with the service in Lewisham was that their midwife was helpful and reassuring. This was reflected in a comment from a Lewisham woman: 'They never make you feel silly. When I had (my son) they made me feel as though I was wasting their time sometimes. Even if I just want reassurance, she'll tell me.' Women valued being treated as individuals and having a service tailored to their needs. Another Lewisham woman felt she was receiving: 'A very personal service – not fronted by a receptionist. It is much less like being part of a herd giving birth. It suits women on their second or third pregnancy because you are not messed around.'

The trusting relationships that developed between women and their midwife was often mentioned and this made women feel confident about the care and advice they were receiving. In contrast, women often referred to the fear that hospital professionals would take over and fail to take their wishes and preferences into account. Some women talked of a feeling of friendship that had developed during the course of pregnancy between themselves and their midwife and was described by a Lewisham woman to be like: 'Having someone you can relate to as a person, like a friend, that I know will be there when I give birth, and she'll respect my wishes when I'm having my baby.'

Women in Ashford valued similar aspects of the service such as helpful and informative midwives and the high standard of care, but also mentioned the value of being cared for by a midwife who was accessible and could be contacted at any time. One woman particularly liked the fact that her midwife spent time at consultations with her: 'It's longer than the time you wait – just the opposite of the hospital.' Other women felt that they were respected and felt more in control in their relationship with their midwives, noting that this was absent in their dealings with hospital staff. A woman in Ashford explained: 'They treat you like an adult, not a child or a patient.' Another woman valued the informality and said of her midwife: 'She didn't have a uniform. That can be quite nice – it's not so starchy.' Another woman said: 'It's a marvellous thing. I'm sorry there are not more of these groups around. I've been lucky, a trouble free pregnancy. I like their attitude that you are not ill; pregnancy is completely normal.' Another woman noted: 'Basically you feel you're having private health care without paying for it.'

A factor which contributed to women's feeling of satisfaction and which was highlighted more in Deptford than elsewhere was that women felt that their choices were respected and they could ask for the care they wanted. A Deptford woman said of her midwife: 'She's taken my wish to have a home birth, even though my first was a breech caesarean. My GP did not have the same response. She indicated that I might have to go into hospital to have the second. She feels that a home birth was not a good idea but X feels quite comfortable with the idea.' Another Deptford woman reflected this view: 'The reassurance that home birth is OK, other people think it's dangerous. With (my last baby) I almost felt as though I was being irresponsible.'

Having choices respected and having someone as an advocate were emphasised by women in Deptford time and time again. One woman said: 'I feel I've got someone on my side, really. Someone I can contact at any time of the day or night about anything. A great relief.' Another woman expressed her satisfaction: 'Because our choices have been completely respected. They really treat you as an individual. We trust her completely and that induces a lot of confidence.' Others talked of the close bond and relationship with their midwife reflected in this comment made by a

Deptford woman: 'It is a close relationship. I think every woman falls in love with her midwife.'

Comparisons with hospital staff often portrayed them as less committed in the eyes of the women than the MGP midwives. A Deptford woman commented about her midwives: 'They're both very understanding of how women feel – they're in tune. I feel they'll respect my wishes more than a midwife at hospital, who might change shift in the middle of labour.'

Women often attributed deficiencies in the service to individuals rather than the system within which hospital staff have to operate. This under-lines the fact that comparisons will inevitably be made between the MGP care and other areas of the service which may be unfair for a variety of reasons. It is important that the good practice which exists in many hospitals should be built upon, but our findings indicate that positive action should be taken to address the concerns about some aspects of hospital-based care which were highlighted by the women we interviewed, both in these first interviews and in the interviews reported in the next chapter. It must also be recognised that hospital staff cannot be expected to provide the same form of care as that provided by the MGPs without the appropriate systems and sufficient resources.

What did women like best about the MGP service?
Determining the level of satisfaction is not in itself sufficient without being able to identify the actual features of the service that women particularly liked or disliked. Many of these factors are important in addressing the question of replicability.

In Lewisham nearly half the women identified home visits as a feature of the service they liked best, reflected in the comments from a Lewisham woman: 'I like the convenience of it. I can be in the comfort of my own home, you're more relaxed at home. Even to give a specimen you can go up to your own loo. It's much nicer. Also with (the midwife) here I feel I can ask more questions. At the clinic you feel you've only got a fifteen minute slot.' Nearly a third of women mentioned the friendliness of the midwives and the positive 'feel good' approach to them and their care. The one-to-one relationship and the continuity of care was endorsed by around a quarter of women and equal emphasis was placed on the person-al service geared to the individual.

In Ashford nearly half the women mentioned the one-to-one relation-ship and continuity of care and between a quarter and a third of women endorsed the personal approach geared to the individual. Nearly a quarter of women mentioned the friendliness and open approach of the midwives reflected in the comment from an Ashford woman: 'You feel welcomed and you can speak freely with her and she'll be straight with you – more like talking to a friend.'

In Deptford 39 per cent of women liked the personal service geared to their needs, and a similar proportion mentioned the trusting relationship with their midwife which was not given the same emphasis elsewhere. One woman described what she liked best about the service: 'The caring approach, genuinely interested in me and my family. For the first time I feel I will be in control at the birth. I have a lot more confidence about the birth to come.' A quarter of women mentioned continuity of care and one woman in Deptford explained how she valued the fact that she would know the midwife attending her in labour: 'I know who the person is going to be. I don't have to worry about some faceless person who doesn't know anything about me.' Equal emphasis was given to the friendliness of the midwives.

What did women like least about the service?

Although many women could not identify anything they did not like about the service and few said they were dissatisfied with it overall, around one third could readily identify a certain aspect of care that they liked least. Some issues were consistently mentioned by women in all areas and should be given further attention.

In Deptford women were likely to mention the uncertainty of the MGP funding as an aspect that they liked least. Other Deptford women said that they did not like the unstructured schedule of antenatal visits. A few women referred to the weak links between the Deptford MGP and local hospitals, particularly in relation to tests, or said that the MGP was too 'politically correct'.

Women in Ashford were more likely than those in other areas to identify an aspect of the service that they liked least, with most of these women mentioning the long gaps between appointments and the unstructured antenatal schedule. In some instances women spoke of feeling neglected or forgotten, as one explained: 'If this was my first baby I'd feel a bit on the neglected side, having such a long gap between appointments.' Another woman said of her midwife: 'I'd have preferred to have seen her more often. After the first consultation I didn't see her for 11 weeks.' Another Ashford woman spoke of the time pressures on the midwives: 'I believe they're under pressure. There aren't enough of them I think. They haven't got enough time for you. I feel the second baby isn't monitored as closely as the first.'

Women in Lewisham were least likely to identify anything they did not like about the service. However, the unstructured antenatal schedule was the most frequently mentioned. A Lewisham woman explained: 'I would like to see her a bit more but she's got a lot to see. She showed me the pack of cases and she has a lot of work.' Lewisham women noted particularly that the midwives seemed to be very busy. One woman said of her midwife: 'I feel she's very rushed. She seems flustered. I suppose she's got a huge workload.' Another Lewisham woman noted: 'Although she listens to me I feel that she's rushing to get on to the next person.' A few women mentioned that they had not received sufficient advice about medical queries or that their midwife had failed to follow up queries and concerns properly. One woman commented: 'I was ill a few weeks ago with a virus and I felt really depressed and worried about the baby maybe having died. She (the midwife) came straight round but there was no follow-up and that would have been nice.'

Women who had received care in previous pregnancies

We have already seen that the MGPs were set up to provide a new form of care that was more accessible, accountable and appropriate to women's needs. The pilot projects aimed to give women increased opportunity to participate in planning and decision making and to increase choice, control and satisfaction.

We asked women in how many of their previous pregnancies they had received midwifery care, whether that care differed from MGP care and in what way. Apart from the women in their first pregnancy, a small proportion of women in all areas (14 per cent in Deptford, 10 per cent in Lewisham and 4 per cent in Ashford) said that they had had previous pregnancies but had not had midwifery care, in most cases because the pregnancy had resulted in a miscarriage or termination of pregnancy. This meant that around two-thirds of women in all areas said that they had received midwifery care in one or more previous pregnancies. (53 per cent of the women interviewed in Deptford, 45 per cent in Ashford and 37 per cent in Lewisham had had midwifery care in one previous pregnancy. 29 per cent of women in Lewisham, 23 per cent in Ashford and 16 per cent in Deptford had had midwifery care in two or more previous pregnancies.) The following discussion relates to women who had received midwifery care in previous pregnancies.

Women in Lewisham were more likely to report that the care in their current pregnancy differed from previous care than women in Deptford or in Ashford. This could have been partly due to the fact that none of the women in Lewisham were receiving care from a midwife whom they already knew from previous pregnancies. 24 per cent of women in Ashford and 17 per cent in Deptford indicated that there was no difference in their care because they were cared for by the same midwife.

Women's current experience of care appeared in some instances to differ fundamentally from the care they had received in the past. Women in all areas consistently identified the personal service provided by the MGPs as a feature of their present care that they had not experienced before. In addition, continuity of care was highlighted by over a quarter of the women in Lewisham and Ashford and by one sixth of the women in Deptford, while increased choice and flexibility was mentioned by a quarter of the women in Lewisham and around one fifth in Deptford and Ashford.

In discussing their previous care, around 40 per cent of women in all three areas referred to the absence of antenatal and intrapartum continuity of care, while around 40 per cent of women in Deptford referred to what they regarded as the impersonal service and clinical emphasis in previous pregnancies, a feature noted by around one fifth of women in the other two areas.

It is noteworthy that, despite the introduction of a new model of care, most women who were treated by the same midwife as in previous pregnancies felt that there was no difference between past and present care. This suggests that some midwives had already moved away from traditional care and that the introduction of the MGP simply formalised practices that were already established. This point is important in relation to the issue of sustainable practice and replicability, because if the new model of care was, in effect, 'more of the same' from a few MGP midwives, it is possible that the model itself may not have been sufficiently tested.

In bidding for inclusion in the pilot project, it is understandable that managers may have chosen a group of motivated midwives who were interested in moving away from traditional approaches to care (or had already done so) in order to increase the MGP's chances of success. Such midwives could also encourage other midwives to change their practice, but the question must be posed of whether these midwives were a representative group. That is not to say that in setting up the MGPs, midwifery managers should not have taken into account the contribution of individual midwives and their willingness to pursue the aims and objectives of the MGP. It may be entirely sensible to choose midwives who are willing and able to demonstrate a particular model of care, but it should also be borne in mind that the midwives who were chosen were already 'converted' and that it may be more difficult to cascade the new way of working across the whole service.

Chapter 6

Women's experience of birth and postnatal care

We interviewed 117 women after their babies were born: 40 in Lewisham, 41 in Ashford and 36 in Deptford. The women were usually interviewed approximately four weeks after the birth of their babies. As we saw in the last chapter, 12 of the 117 women had not been interviewed before their babies were born, mainly because they had booked or transferred at a late stage in their pregnancies to the midwifery group practices. Six of these women had booked with or transferred to the MGPs in April or July 1995 but had delivered their babies before we could conduct a first interview with them. Otherwise, all the women had booked with or transferred to the MGPs in the first four sampling periods: April, July and October 1994 and January 1995.

There were some differences between the areas in the months in which the babies were born. This appears to have been mainly due to the fact that women in Ashford booked at an earlier stage in their pregnancies with the MGP than in the other areas, so that we interviewed them for the first time earlier in their pregnancies. Around two-thirds of the babies in Lewisham and Deptford were born in the period between September 1994 and March 1995, compared with just over 50 per cent of the babies in Ashford, while around one third in Lewisham and Deptford were born between April and September 1995 compared with just under half of the Ashford babies.

We are therefore looking at the experience of women who had booked with the group practices during the monitoring period and had had their babies under the care of the MGP midwives. However, the length of their antenatal care from the MGP midwives varied widely, as we saw in the last chapter and in Chapter 3.

The babies

65 per cent of the babies in Lewisham were girls, compared with 51 per cent in Ashford and 47 per cent in Deptford. One set of twins was born in Lewisham.

First babies accounted for 28 per cent (11) of the Lewisham babies, 25 per cent (9) of the Deptford babies and 41 per cent (17) of the Ashford babies. This meant, of course, that the women we interviewed had rather more previous experience of childbirth than we would expect in a completely representative national sample of women having babies. Two-thirds of all the women had had at least one baby before, but the distribution was slightly skewed, with three-quarters of the Lewisham and Deptford women and 59 per cent of the Ashford women having had a baby before. In the total sample of 180 women with whom we conducted interviews (see Table 5.7) the distribution was more even among the areas, with two-thirds in all areas having had at least one baby already. The slight differences may be accounted for by the changes which took place in the clientele of the Ashford MGP over the period: for example, the earlier bookings in Ashford included all risk categories. But it is more likely that the pattern of one third first babies: two-thirds second or subsequent babies is a more accurate reflection of the profile of women using the MGPs.

Location and type of birth
There were marked differences between the areas in the location of births of the babies.

Home births
- 18 per cent (7) of the Lewisham babies were born at home
- 10 per cent (4) of the Ashford babies were born at home
- 64 per cent (23) of the Deptford babies were born at home

Hospital births
- 82 per cent (33) of the Lewisham babies were born at Lewisham Hospital
- 90 per cent (37) of the Ashford babies were born at William Harvey Hospital
- 36 per cent (13) of the Deptford babies were born in hospital:
  - 11 per cent (4) in Lewisham Hospital
  - 19 per cent (7) in King's College Hospital
  - 6 per cent (2) in Greenwich Hospital

But was this where the women had planned to have their babies?
- Of the 34 women who had home births, 31 had planned to have their babies at home but 3 had planned to have them in hospital.
- Of the 83 who had their babies in hospital, on the other hand, 68 (82 per cent) had planned this; 13 women (16 per cent) had planned a home birth but had had a hospital birth instead; 2 had had no definite plans before labour.

Looking specifically at the 13 women from all Mgps who had planned a home birth but had had a hospital birth, it was perhaps not surprising that 10 of these women were with the Deptford MGP, given their interest in home births.

Only 4 of the 36 women cared for by the Deptford MGP had planned hospital births: of these, 3 had hospital births and 1 had a home birth. But what this means is that 10 of the 13 Deptford women who had hospital births had planned home births. This was true of only 2 women in Lewisham and 1 woman in Ashford.

Why was there a change of plan from home to hospital? In just under a quarter of cases, the baby was in a breech position; in the same proportion of cases, the labour was painful and the woman wanted greater pain control; in the same proportion of cases the labour was long and slow, while in slightly fewer cases a caesarean birth was found necessary. One woman became afraid of a home birth, another changed her mind just before she went into labour, while in another case the consultant advised a hospital birth because of the large size of the baby.

Of the three who changed from hospital to home births, one had a very quick labour and did not have time to get to hospital, one chose to change because a normal birth was predicted, while the other changed her mind shortly before the expected date of delivery.

On the whole the women were not concerned at the change of place of delivery or accepted that it was necessary for the safety of the baby or themselves. All of them felt that they had had enough discussion of the change of location of the birth.

Type of delivery

What kind of delivery did the women have?
* *spontaneous vaginal delivery:*
  78 per cent Lewisham and Deptford; 73 per cent Ashford
* *induced vaginal delivery:*
  5 per cent Lewisham; 5 per cent Deptford; 20 per cent Ashford
* *instrumental:*
  5 per cent Lewisham; 8 per cent Deptford; none in Ashford
* *emergency caesarean:*
  5 per cent Lewisham and Ashford; 8 per cent Deptford
* *elective caesarean:*
  8 per cent Lewisham; 5 per cent Ashford; 3 per cent Deptford

Professionals present during labour

The extent to which the woman's named midwife was present during her labour varied, as Table 6.1 shows. In Lewisham, the named midwife was present in 61 per cent of cases, compared with 51 per cent in Ashford but as many as 92 per cent in Deptford. Another MGP midwife was present at 40 per cent of labours in Lewisham, 44 per cent in Ashford and 72 per cent in Deptford.

Table 6.1   Professionals present during labour

column percentages

	Lewisham	Ashford	Deptford
Named midwife	61	51	92
Another MGP midwife	40	44	72
Hospital midwife	13	37	6
Student/placement MW	5	24	6
Consultant obstetrician(s)	3	0	6
Other hospital doctor(s)	13	39	14
GP	0	2	0
Anaesthetist	3	7	6
Paediatrician	3	2	0
Nobody	0	0	3
No labour	8	5	3
Base: all women	*(40)*	*(41)*	*(36)*

The table shows quite a marked difference between Ashford and the other areas, with 37 per cent of the Ashford women having a hospital midwife and 24 per cent a student midwife present during labour, compared with far fewer of these in both Lewisham and Deptford. Similarly, a hospital doctor other than a consultant was present during labour in 39 per cent of cases in Ashford, compared with just over 10 per cent in both Lewisham and Deptford.

When we analysed the figures in more detail, we found that the different pattern of working by the MGPs that had emerged in Chapters 2, 3 and 4 was highlighted in these interviews.

• In Lewisham, the most common pattern was for the woman to be seen in labour either by her named midwife alone (38 per cent), another MGP midwife alone (28 per cent) or by her named midwife and a hospital midwife (13 per cent). This accounted for 80 per cent of cases. Only in 8 per cent of cases was a woman in labour seen by her named midwife *and* another MGP midwife.

• In Ashford, it was unusual for a woman to be seen in labour by her named midwife alone (20 per cent), or by another MGP midwife alone (2 per cent), or by her named midwife and a hospital midwife (5 per cent). This only amounted to 27 per cent compared with nearly 80 per cent in Lewisham. In 19 per cent of cases another MGP midwife attended in labour with a hospital or student midwife. In 12 per cent of cases a woman in labour was seen by her named midwife *and* another MGP midwife.

• In Deptford, the pattern was completely different. It was unusual for a woman to be seen in labour by her named midwife alone (19 per cent) or another MGP midwife alone (3 per cent), but 61 per cent were seen by both the named midwife *and* another MGP midwife. One woman was seen by nobody during her labour and one was seen by a named midwife and a hospital midwife.

How much did it matter to the women that their named midwife was present during labour? We have seen that this happened in almost all the cases in Deptford, but in 60 per cent of cases in Lewisham and just over half the cases in Ashford. Most women whose named midwife was present said that it mattered a lot to them that she was there, but one in ten of the Lewisham women said that it did not matter at all, and one fifth of the Ashford women said that it mattered, but not a lot.

The main reasons for women wanting their named midwife present during labour was that she offered reassurance, increased their confidence, gave security and provided familiarity. The women to whom it mattered a lot were often overwhelming in their praise, like a Lewisham woman: 'I don't think I could have got through without her. I really trusted her – she knew what I wanted and what I didn't want in labour. She knew what I was worried about as well. I trusted her more than the doctors.' Trust was clearly a keynote with some women, and was mentioned by a Deptford woman in a different context: 'I have absolute trust in her and she trusts me. She understood where I was coming from. I knew she wouldn't interfere unnecessarily.'

However, some women were not particularly concerned about whether their named midwife was there or not, like a woman in Lewisham: 'Quite honestly, with my other births I didn't have a named midwife and it didn't really make a lot of difference.'

What about those whose named midwife was not present during their labour? What did they feel about the lack of continuity of carer during their labour? The women were perhaps surprisingly unperturbed, and less than one in ten (all in Ashford) said that they were disappointed, although two women (both in Ashford) said that they were disappointed for the midwife – 'It didn't matter for me at all in the end. I was disappointed for her rather than me because she was on holiday.'

On the whole, the women said that the reasons had been explained, or that they had met the other MGP midwives, or that they were happy with the hospital midwives. In Ashford, an underlying theme in some of the interviews both during the pregnancy and after the delivery was the perceived infrequency of consultations with midwives in any case, as this woman pointed out: 'I didn't mind because I hadn't seen much of them. I had a bit of a problem with them – I only saw them a few times. They never did the birth plan, so eventually I called them. I kept asking to be put into the classes and then one said, "You've missed them now."'

Sometimes things went wrong, and the extent to which the Lewisham system of concentrating care of the woman with the MGP without sufficient apparent liaison with the hospital could lead to unhappy experiences was highlighted by this woman: 'I tried to contact (named midwife) at 6 am when labour started and I couldn't get hold of her. I rang the ambulance at 7 am. I then phoned (other MGP midwife). She said she would meet me at the hospital. When I arrived at the hospital there was no-one there. I was told to go to the labour ward and nobody showed me to the ward, and I sat alone in a room. I arrived in the hospital at about 7.30 am. At about 7.45 a hospital midwife came on duty and when she checked me I was 7 cm dilated. I couldn't believe it. It was terrible. Nobody even helped me with my bags. I was just told to go to room 7.'

Other people present during labour

In over 90 per cent of cases other friends or relatives were present during the woman's labour. In the vast majority of cases the woman's husband or partner was present, although this was rather less common in Deptford than in the other areas. Friends were present with nearly one third of the Deptford women, compared with around one in ten of the other women. Mothers and sisters were more likely to be present with Lewisham and Ashford women than the Deptford women, but perhaps it is a sign of the times that mothers were present at less than one in five of labours, even in Lewisham.

On the whole the women had planned for their labour companions to be present, although some said that they had planned for some but not others. One woman in Lewisham knew that her husband was unlikely to be a willing participant: 'My husband had wanted to be absent from the gory bits. He's been put off by videos at the antenatal classes. But he was at home throughout the labour and got involved.'

Preparation for labour

Careful preparation of women for labour and delivery is clearly a crucial part of antenatal care, and was stressed by all the MGPs as part of their interpretation of *Changing Childbirth*. It must also be remembered that a high proportion of these women had had previous births, so that it might be thought that most would be well prepared in any case.

It was therefore surprising to find that over one third of the women in Lewisham and Ashford and over one fifth of the Deptford women said that they were not prepared for everything that happened to them during labour.

Women felt unprepared for quite a variety of things, but the main features were long, difficult or painful labours, (mentioned by one third of those who were unprepared), and speed of labour or other complications (each mentioned by one fifth of those who were unprepared). In addition, women mentioned being unprepared for emergency caesareans, epidurals, induction, episiotomies, foetal distress and premature births.

It would be expected that all of these possible features of childbirth would be mentioned by midwives in the antenatal period. Perhaps the feeling of lack of preparation for what happened expressed by these women is part of the 'it won't happen to me' syndrome that many people adopt in relation to a wide variety of things in life, including, of course, getting pregnant in the first place.

But there were also other matters that women felt unprepared for which related to the organisation of the MGPs. Two women in different areas were concerned that there was only one midwife in attendance and another was concerned that no MGP midwife was present.

The question of how to prepare women for pain or complications in labour or delivery is not new, but clearly the MGPs were not always any more successful than other professionals before them. Many of the comments from women could have illustrated the practices the MGPs were trying hard to eradicate. A woman in Lewisham said: 'They didn't tell me her heartbeat was dropping. They put me on a drip which slowed the heartbeat. It could have been dealt with better. They weren't explaining things to me or to my husband as they happened. We didn't know what was going on.'

Another Lewisham woman felt unprepared for complications: 'It would have been nice if they had talked about different types of birth beforehand. All the classes were about normal births.' An Ashford woman wanted: '...more information about everything from start to finish. I just wanted some sort of explanation – like how would I know when labour had started?'

In some cases there appears to have been a breakdown in care, most dramatically highlighted in Ashford: 'I had a three month gap between appointments with the group practice midwives – between the end of October and mid January. If I'd had one, they'd have discovered that I had diabetes and I would have been prepared. It's a miracle that I didn't die at Christmas – all the sweets I ate – two packets of Roses.'

When we asked the women how they felt they could have been better prepared, around half of them were fairly philosophical and said that it was difficult to say how they could have been better prepared. Others were not so sanguine and there were murmurs of discontent with the preparation they received.

Pain control

There were marked differences between the areas in the forms of pain control used by the women during labour, some of which were clearly related to the differences in the place of birth.

In Deptford, nearly 40 per cent of the women said that they had *no pain control* in labour, compared with around one fifth of the women in both Lewisham and Ashford. On the other hand, 28 per cent of the Deptford women used *water,* compared with 5 per cent in Ashford and none in Lewisham.

Nearly two-thirds of the Lewisham and Ashford women used *Entonox,* compared with a quarter of the Deptford women. One in six of the women in all areas used TENS. One fifth of the Lewisham women, nearly one third of the Ashford women but no Deptford women had a *pethidine injection.*

One in ten of the Lewisham and Deptford women had an *epidural* compared with one in six in Ashford. Massage and homeopathy were mentioned by three women.

But did the pain control meet their needs? For most women it did, but nearly one fifth of the Lewisham women, over one in ten of the Ashford women and a quarter of the Deptford women said that it did not. The reasons were mainly related to the strength of the pain, but in Ashford there was a disturbing account from one respondent, highlighting again the potential dangers when MGP patients are seen as 'different' from the mainstream: 'I'd requested some kind of painkiller when I was on the labour ward, but I didn't get anything until two hours later when (MGP midwife) arrived. I was disgusted with that. But all I got from the midwives in hospital is that "we shouldn't be seeing you because you're with the JACANES group".'

In Deptford pain control did not meet one woman's needs for another reason: 'The pool collapsed and we had 150 gallons of water in the house. She called the other midwives and they sorted it out. They piled up the furniture and got rid of all the water. It was just incredible.'

It appears that midwives may need a variety of skills in extending the frontiers of their practice.

Physical and emotional needs in labour

Apart from pain control, we were interested in the extent to which women felt that their physical and emotional needs were met during their labour. Around 90 per cent of the women said that their physical needs were met. The care was generally thought to be good, and some women commented on the differences between their care on this occasion and previous occasions.

A Deptford woman valued the freedom she was given by the midwife: 'When I wanted to go for a bath I could. I didn't have those awful internal examinations. She was brilliant. There was none of this "Do you think you should do this?" She did not interfere. In the hospital I had to fight with the midwife for a pillow. The midwife would not kneel down because she did not want to hurt her back.'

Over 80 per cent of the Lewisham and Ashford women and over 90 per cent of the Deptford women said that their emotional needs were met during labour. An Ashford woman said: 'My husband was very emotional too and we were allowed to have a good old sob.'

The few women with complaints about emotional needs often related them to lack of pain relief or lack of reassurance or not knowing what was happening. However, again, there were indications that not all practice was of the high standards expected: 'I kept wanting more reassurance. I didn't know if I was breathing the gas and air properly. She just said, "Breathe naturally." And she kept going off for a nap. I sent my husband to find her a couple of times. It was horrible actually.'

In other instances, the unpredictability of childbirth might have been a factor: 'I was scared and at the time I haemorrhaged I was left with the trainee. I felt so sorry for her – it was awful for her. The doctors were just doing their rounds then, so they came in and sorted everything out.'

The overwhelming majority of women in all areas felt that they had enough privacy during labour, and interestingly the main complaints were levelled at friends and relatives coming in uninvited.

Professionals present during delivery

We have already seen that there were marked differences between the areas in the extent to which different professionals were present during labour, and these were found again when we asked who was present at delivery.

Table 6.2 shows that the named midwife was present at 92 per cent of the births in Deptford, compared with 71 per cent in Lewisham and 49 per cent in Ashford. Another MGP midwife was present at 75 per cent of the births in Deptford, 55 per cent in Lewisham and 41 per cent in Ashford. It should be noted that in one case in Deptford, no professional was present, either during labour or at delivery.

The striking difference between Ashford and the other two areas in the presence of hospital or student midwives was noteworthy again at delivery, with 37 per cent of the Ashford births attended by a hospital midwife and 20 per cent by a student midwife, compared with around 10 per cent attended by hospital midwives in Lewisham and Deptford and few student midwives in either area.

Similarly, hospital doctors other than consultants were much more likely to be present at delivery in Ashford (32 per cent) than in Lewisham (18 per cent) or Deptford (17 per cent).

Table 6.2   Professionals present during delivery

column percentages

	Lewisham	Ashford	Deptford
Named midwife	71	49	92
Another MGP midwife	55	41	75
Hospital midwife	10	37	14
Student/placement MW	8	20	6
Consultant obstetrician(s)	13	2	11
Other hospital doctor(s)	18	32	17
GP	0	2	3
Anaesthetist	8	10	11
Paediatrician	13	12	8
Nobody	0	0	3
Base: all women	*(40)*	*(41)*	*(36)*

Although the proportions of hospital midwives and doctors present at delivery look much the same for Lewisham and Deptford, it should be remembered that a much lower proportion of Deptford deliveries were in hospital than in Lewisham. There are clear indications that the Lewisham MGP midwives took on the role of hospital midwives to a much greater extent than the Deptford midwives when their patients gave birth in hospital.

The pattern of practice noted before is reinforced when we analysed the figures further.

- In 56 per cent of Deptford cases, the named midwife *and* another MGP midwife were present at delivery, compared with 23 per cent of cases in Lewisham and only 12 per cent in Ashford.

- In 36 per cent of cases in Lewisham, the named midwife was present at delivery as the only midwife, compared with 25 per cent in Ashford and 17 per cent in Deptford. (In a small number of cases in all three areas doctors were also present.)

- In 25 per cent of cases in Lewisham, another MGP midwife was present at delivery as the only midwife, compared with 10 per cent in Ashford and 6 per cent in Deptford. (Again, in a small number of cases in all three areas doctors were also present.)

- In 22 per cent of Ashford cases, hospital midwives were present at delivery *without* an MGP midwife, with or without hospital doctors. This did not occur in either of the other areas.

Essentially, the figures show how impossible it was for the Ashford MGP midwives to guarantee their presence at delivery for the enormous number of women they were booking in the first twelve months of the monitoring period.

Views on presence or absence of named midwife at delivery

We asked the women whose named midwife was present at delivery how much it mattered to them. All but one of the Deptford women said that it mattered a lot, but this was only true of three-quarters of the Lewisham and Ashford women. The main reasons the women gave for appreciating the presence of their named midwife at delivery were the same as those given for her presence during labour – to give reassurance, confidence, security and to provide familiarity and friendliness. Around a fifth of the women whose named midwife was present said that they liked the continuity of carer, while over a quarter of the Deptford women, most of whom had their babies at home, said that they appreciated the professional skills of the midwives and their readiness to take responsibility if a problem occurred.

Some of the comments from women in all areas showed the enormous rapport which had been built up between the midwives and the women. A Lewisham woman was eloquent in her praise: 'I knew she really cared about me. I trusted her and I knew she wouldn't do anything she didn't have to. And I knew she really loved children. She's so dedicated. She was so calm and reassuring. She'd been up all day Tuesday. She made me comfortable in hospital and she was gone an hour. She was up with me all Tuesday night – all Wednesday. I had the baby on Wednesday afternoon. She was exhausted – smiling and laughing – really caring. All the time she was in hospital – Tuesday night to Wednesday afternoon – she had to keep going out to put money in the meter so her car wouldn't be clamped. The car park is owned by a private company and they don't care. And she never ate anything all that time.'

This quote is presented in its entirety, because it says a great deal, not only about the quality of the relationship and the care given by the midwife, but also about the conditions under which she was working and the dedication which she, but perhaps not everyone, was prepared to give to the job.

Familiarity was clearly important to some women. An Ashford woman noted: 'I trusted her totally. Whatever she said I did. When you're on gas and air you get a bit sky-high. I knew her voice.' Another woman in Ashford also stressed the importance she attached to a known person: 'It makes all the difference having a woman that you know, rather than a stranger. It's a worse affront to think that the world at large has seen all your most private places.'

And trust in midwives was sometimes total, as a woman in Deptford explained: 'I would do anything she told me to do – even stand on my head.'

The women who were less concerned about the presence of their midwives mainly said that they would have been happy with other midwives or that they were in too much pain or distress to care who was present, like a woman in Lewisham: 'I didn't mind. When you are delivering you don't mind if the man down the shop delivers you, once the pain is there.'

Of the women whose named midwife was not present at the delivery, the vast majority were happy with the care they received from other midwives. Only 4 women (all in Ashford) said that they were disappointed in that they would have liked continuity of carer, while 3 women said that they were disappointed for the midwife's sake that she was not there.

Other people present during delivery

95 per cent of the women interviewed said that a relative or friend was present during delivery, with virtually the same proportion in each area. The woman's husband or partner was present in around 80 per cent of cases where someone else was present, although this was rather less frequent in Lewisham than in the other two areas. Mothers and sisters were present in around one in ten deliveries. In Deptford, friends were there in nearly a quarter of cases where someone else was present, but much less often in the other two areas, probably because home births were more frequent in Deptford. Children were present in 6 per cent of the Deptford births, but not at all in the other two areas.

In most cases the women had planned for the presence of the relatives or friends at the birth, but some had not planned for everyone who came, one or two of whom had 'just turned up', and one husband who had originally not intended to be there because he was 'squeamish', but evidently could not drag himself away at the end.

Preparation for delivery

The women appeared rather better prepared for delivery than for labour, although some seemed surprisingly ill-prepared. 81 per cent of the Deptford women, 73 per cent of the Lewisham women and 66 per cent of the Ashford women said that they were prepared for everything that happened to them at delivery.

In fact, the most frequent source of surprise in each area was the speed of the delivery, mentioned by one third of the women who felt unprepared. One in six felt unprepared for the degree of pain they experienced. Others mentioned the shock of foetal distress, having a forceps delivery, being cut or tearing, an emergency caesarean, an epidural, an induction, the length of time the delivery took, and other complications. One Deptford woman was taken completely by surprise: 'Labour and delivery were so fast. I had planned to have a waterbirth, but I didn't have time to get into the pool.'

Most women who said that they were unprepared for certain aspects of their delivery said that they probably could not have been better prepared, given the circumstances, although a small number thought that more written information or attendance at antenatal classes would have helped. Some were relieved that they had not been fully prepared, like an Ashford woman who had a forceps delivery when her baby went into distress: 'I don't think I could have been better prepared. I don't think I would have wanted that explained to me beforehand, and because I didn't know I didn't worry.'

Pain control

The Deptford women again used least pain control. 58 per cent of them said that they used *no pain control in delivery,* compared with 30 per cent in Lewisham and 22 per cent in Ashford. Even allowing for the small numbers, the differences in the use of pain control at delivery were marked. For example, nearly 60 per cent in Lewisham used *Entonox,* compared with 44 per cent in Ashford and 8 per cent in Deptford. 14 per cent of the Deptford women had a *waterbirth,* compared with 2 per cent in Ashford and none in Lewisham. Around one in six of the Lewisham and Ashford women had an *epidural* compared with one in ten in Deptford. Very few women in any area used TENS at delivery. *Pethidine* was used by over one in ten in Lewisham and Ashford, but by no-one in Deptford. Two women spoke of having a general anaesthetic.

In nearly 90 per cent of the cases where women used pain relief they said it met their needs. Some appeared to overdo it: 'I had Entonox – I bit it to pieces. They can't use it again.'

Physical and emotional needs at delivery

All but one woman interviewed said that all their physical needs were met during delivery. The only exception said that her bladder was perforated during delivery and she had had to have it repaired and to be catheterised for nine days after delivery.

The overwhelming majority of women said that all their emotional needs were met during delivery, and the only problems appeared to occur when the baby was in distress at birth.

Hospital and home births

The debate over home and hospital births is often conducted by strong proponents of one view or the other. But what did the women who were interviewed think? We asked the women what they liked most and what they liked least about giving birth in the place that they had their babies.

Hospital births

Nearly 90 per cent of the Lewisham and Ashford women who gave birth in hospital said that they liked most the feeling of security and safety given by hospital births, a view shared by just over two-thirds of the Deptford women who gave birth in hospital. However, nearly a quarter of the Deptford women said that the pain relief was what they liked most about the hospital birth, compared with less than one in ten of the others.

Other factors were mentioned by a handful of women in each area, including good food, pleasant surroundings, rest, privacy, a birthing pool, nice hospital midwives and having a normal delivery. However, four women – two each in Lewisham and Deptford said that there was nothing they liked about having a hospital birth.

Women were often enthusiastic about the surroundings, and some of the descriptions sounded very cosy: 'I hadn't imagined a room to myself. It had a big old-fashioned rocking chair and it was really nice. And I had tea and toast afterwards with strawberry jam.' Others described the hospital like a hotel – '...and I've been in some of the best hotels in the world...' – while others liked – '...the constant attention. There's always something going on and you get treated really well.'

One of the few Deptford women who had her baby in hospital was quite clear about her preference: 'It's in my mind that if something goes wrong, everything is there. And at home there is a mess and you might disturb neighbours by screaming. In the hospital, I felt free to scream and I was more relaxed.'

However, although 40 per cent of the women who had had hospital births said that there was nothing they disliked about the experience, others had complaints. The surroundings, the lack of comfort and the lack of privacy were mentioned most frequently by Lewisham and Deptford women. Some criticisms were very sharp – '...the postnatal ward is filthy – the bathrooms and things – there is no excuse...' However, other women in each area found the hospital ambience too clinical and technological.

There were disquieting signs throughout these interviews that in both Lewisham and Ashford there was little communication between the midwifery group practices and the hospital midwives, with the result that some of the women we interviewed reported unhappy accounts of what amounted to neglect and rudeness from hospital staff. A Lewisham woman gave a graphic account of her treatment: 'Everyone ignored me. I always had to ask for things. I had to ask for painkillers. When leaving I had to carry my two bags, my baby and myself the whole way down through casualty. I had to wait one hour for a cab. Before, with my previous pregnancy (elsewhere) that did not happen. The nurses helped me carry my baby and bags... I thought that maybe because I was on the scheme they were giving me no attention. I felt very neglected in that hospital. No-one else in there was on the scheme and I think that was the reason.'

Another woman in Lewisham agreed: 'There was no-one to look after me after the delivery. I went to the ward and the first time I saw anyone was when I asked if I could go home 48 hours later.' Her experience was echoed by another woman: 'I wasn't happy after the birth. Once (MGP midwife) had gone I was left to it. The paediatrician had been to see me and I was told I would have to wait a day. Nobody brought me a meal. I had to keep asking various people what was happening – when I could go home. They had forgotten about me.'

It did appear that women in both Lewisham and Ashford were regarded as being outside the system in some way. Many of the accounts illustrated what can only be described as bad practice. In Ashford one woman said: 'They don't help. They walk past you. There was no help on things like feeding. I was in hospital three nights and I didn't know how to change nappies, but they didn't help.' Her experience was shared in Lewisham: 'They kept me in hospital for one night and I didn't like it in the ward at all. I didn't get any help at all. I've never had a baby before. I didn't know how to do a nappy and I was having problems with the feeding. Nobody offered to help.'

Some women noted more overt tension between the hospital midwives and the midwifery group practices: 'The hospital midwives don't seem to have a good word for the JACANES group.' But in some cases the lack of communication between professionals was much more potentially danger-ous: 'None of the staff in the maternity ward knew about my diabetes. They gave me treacle tart for dinner. The doctors in the diabetic unit were brilliant – but there was no communication with the maternity staff.'

Home births

The main thing that women liked about giving birth at home was that they were in familiar surroundings and their own bed. This was mentioned by all the women in Lewisham and Ashford who had a home birth and by three-quarters of the Deptford women. The second most important factor was having family and children around them, mentioned by nearly half the women having home births. Other important factors were not having to travel to hospital, privacy and feeling in control. For a quarter of the women in Deptford the lack of drugs or other interventions was the most important factor, although this was hardly mentioned by other women.

The lack of interruption to family life was an interesting feature of some of these interviews, as a Deptford woman explained: 'It was part of my life at home. It was like a normal day except I had a baby in the evening and I had dinner and a bath and I went up to bed in my own bed and the next day life carried on.'

A number of women spoke of the sense of calmness they felt at home – something which they clearly felt to be lacking in hospital. A Lewisham woman said: 'I didn't have to think of anything. I had access to food, drink and my own clothes. I had music on and incense burning. It was being in my own environment. It was all very calm.' And an Ashford woman agreed: 'It was the sense of peace and calm and privacy. It was almost like being in a dream. It was very hot and we were able to open the windows. It was the middle of the night and it was just so tranquil. And just being able to hold him. Then the midwife said she'd make a cup of tea and she left us alone. Then she came up with the tea and it was just like silver service.'

Others described a sense of naturalness and normality – 'It was just like a family party and it just felt right...'

Many of these accounts must be seen in juxtaposition with the accounts of hospital treatment in the last section. The desire for home births may well be related to previous experience of hospitals rather than based on a balanced assessment of the options. The desire for peaceful and tranquil surroundings and atmosphere may well outweigh the risks in the minds of women and this should be taken into account by those responsible for maternity services.

Again, however, there were complaints about home births, even if half the women could think of nothing they disliked. Around one in six of the women found their home births anything but tranquil in that they were expected to continue with the domestic chores and not have a rest. Around one in ten complained about the number of visitors and calls they had. And one in ten complained about the mess: 'The sofa was ruined...'

Postnatal care

We were interested in establishing from whom the women thought they could get help and support after the baby was born, and who had told them about these sources of help.

The overwhelming majority of women in all areas said that they knew what help and support they could expect from their *midwife* after the baby was born. They mostly said that they knew this from their named midwife, but a few knew it from previous experience or from other professionals.

Far fewer said that they knew what they could expect from their *GPs,* but there were differences in the areas, with 78 per cent in Ashford saying they knew what help and support they would get from their GPs, compared with 56 per cent in Deptford and 50 per cent in Lewisham. Again the main source of information was their named midwife, followed by previous experience. Only around one in ten of the Lewisham and Ashford women said that their GPs had told them what help they could expect from them, compared with one fifth of the Deptford women.

Around 90 per cent of the women said that they knew what help and support they would receive from their *health visitors*. In Ashford this information had mainly come from the midwives, but this had happened in only one third of the cases in Lewisham and Deptford, where women were more likely to base their knowledge on previous experience.

Postnatal care from named midwife

Almost all the Lewisham and Deptford women felt that help and advice were readily available from their named midwife, but one in six of the Ashford women did not, mainly because their midwife was on holiday or covering for sick colleagues.

Most of the comments on the immediate postnatal care received from the named midwives were positive, and some underlined the close relationships already established. A Lewisham woman said: 'I was quite upset when she signed me off. She'd become a friend. I was choked.' And another Lewisham woman underlined the dedication to the job that some of the midwives had: 'She came in at 7.30 in the morning. I was so surprised. She'd left me at 5.30 in the afternoon. She said she'd given her kids £20 to spend at McDonald and gone straight to bed and slept through to half past six in the morning.'

The main aspect of the postnatal care that the women liked was that the midwife was always available when needed. In some cases this was very frequent, and the 28-day postnatal care offered as a matter of course by the Deptford midwives was clearly of great comfort to some women: 'I was phoning her all the time. I had problems with breastfeeding. I had mastitis and they were very good. They phoned the doctor, got antibiotics for me, got a breast pump for me. They put me in contact with a breast-feeding counsellor. I phoned them every day for a month. I would say they were glad to discharge me.'

Infant feeding

Over 90 per cent of the women in Lewisham and Deptford said that their named midwives had offered them information and advice about infant feeding. One in ten of the Ashford women said that they had not been offered this advice, mainly because their midwives were on holiday or unavailable at the time.

There were differences between the areas in when the women had discussed infant feeding with their midwives. Half the Deptford women and one third of the Lewisham and Ashford women said they had been offered information and advice *both antenatally and postnatally*. Around 40 per cent in Lewisham and Deptford and a quarter in Ashford said that the advice had been given *postnatally only*. Around 40 per cent in Ashford, a quarter in Lewisham and just over 10 per cent in Deptford said it had been offered *antenatally only*.

We asked the women about the outcome of the advice and information. 83 per cent of the Deptford women said that they then breastfed only,

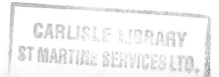

compared with 38 per cent in Lewisham and 39 per cent in Ashford. 38 per cent in Lewisham, 33 per cent in Ashford but only 3 per cent in Deptford were bottlefeeding only. A small proportion in all areas mixed breastfeeding and bottlefeeding, while around one fifth of the women in Lewisham and Ashford breastfed initially and then bottlefed, compared with only 6 per cent in Deptford.

The Deptford midwives certainly achieved very high breastfeeding rates among the women we interviewed in comparison with those in other areas. The women indicated that the midwives showed great interest in maintaining breastfeeding. One Deptford woman said: 'I'm sure their advice and guidance made it very clean and easy. The support is just so strong. There is hardly anyone I know who isn't breastfeeding and I'm sure that is because of the midwives.'

There were some indications in all areas that the women had mixed advice from professionals. An Ashford woman hoped to breastfeed for six months, but pointed up problems: 'The health visitor's advice differed from the midwife's. I wish they'd get together and share a common policy.' And a Deptford woman said: 'At the hospital they were appalling. Each person would give you different advice. They weren't really supportive of breastfeeding. They'd bring bottles and the temptation was enormous, despite the fact that I wanted to breastfeed. I don't think they have their policy sorted out at the hospital.'

Length and frequency of MGP postnatal care

How long did the women continue to see the midwife postnatally?

- In Ashford, 50 per cent of the women saw their midwives for ten days, compared with 40 per cent in Lewisham and only 6 per cent in Deptford.

- In Deptford, on the other hand, 50 per cent of the women saw their midwives for 28 days, compared with 15 per cent in Lewisham and none in Ashford.

- Just over one third of the Lewisham and Ashford women saw their midwives for between 10 and 28 days, compared with 14 per cent in Deptford.

- 5 per cent of the Ashford and Lewisham women said that they saw their midwives for less than 10 days.

- 31 per cent of the Deptford women saw their midwives for more than 28 days, compared with none in the other two areas.

This analysis shows the enormous difference in practice between the Deptford MGP and the others, with 81 per cent of the women we interviewed saying that they saw their midwives for 28 days or longer post-natally, compared with none in Ashford and 15 per cent in Lewisham.

But how often did they see the midwives? We have seen in Chapter 4 that, although the Deptford midwives discharged the women at a much later stage than the other MGPs, the average number of visits was not markedly different.

Well over half the Deptford women said that they initially saw the midwife every day and then less frequently, compared with around a quarter of the women in the other two areas. One third of the Lewisham women said that they had seen the midwife every day – usually for ten days – compared with just over 10 per cent in Ashford and none in Deptford.

The longer the women had seen the midwives the more likely they were to say that they had seen them frequently but not daily – reported by one in five of the Lewisham women, a quarter in Ashford and over one third in Deptford.

However, one fifth of the Lewisham women and over one third of the Ashford women said that they had had fewer than five visits from the mid-wives, compared with only two of the Deptford women.

In addition, nearly 90 per cent of women in Lewisham and Deptford and 75 per cent in Ashford received postnatal care from other midwives, usually other members of the MGPs. Most women could not remember how often this happened.

The main points to come from this analysis were the difficulty in assessing the frequency or intensity of postnatal midwifery care from statistical evidence alone, since so much depended on whether the birth was a home or hospital birth, the length of hospital stay, and the condition of both mother and baby. It was also clear that women could not remember exactly how often they saw the midwives in the postnatal period.

It was quite clear, however, that the Deptford midwives were much more likely than the others to be visiting for much longer postnatally and that their visits were thought to be frequent. The extent to which their visits and duties overlapped with those of health visitors was not explored by us in these interviews, but there seemed to be ample room for duplication of effort and potential conflict of responsibilities.

Women's views on the midwifery group practice

We used a variety of methods of exploring the women's views and experience of the midwifery group practices. We asked them first about their positive memories of the pregnancy and birth and asked whether and how the midwife had contributed to these.

Positive memories of pregnancy and birth

The women had a wide variety of positive memories. Interestingly no one factor was reported by more than a quarter of the women in any one area.

- The most frequently mentioned positive memory in each area was the good standard of individual and personal care given by the midwife – cited by a quarter of the Lewisham women and one fifth of the Deptford and Ashford women.

- The second most frequently mentioned positive memory was of a normal or quick delivery – cited by a quarter of women in Ashford, one fifth in Lewisham but less than 10 per cent in Deptford.

- A healthy trouble-free pregnancy was mentioned by over a quarter of Ashford women, one fifth in Deptford but only by one Lewisham woman.

Other factors relating to the midwifery group practices reported by more than 10 per cent of women in each area were the friendliness of the midwives, the accessibility of the midwives, and the continuity of carer – mentioned by a quarter of the Lewisham women.

Other positive memories of the pregnancy and birth were, not surprisingly, personal to the women themselves, and included feeling the baby moving, the actual delivery of the baby, feeling 'special' during the pregnancy and birth, having more visitors than usual, having the family involved, feeling in control and experiencing personal development through the pregnancy and birth.

When we asked the women what they enjoyed most about the pregnancy and birth, the personal elements were clearly the most important factors. One third said that they most enjoyed the arrival of the baby – or the end of their pregnancy – and one in six most enjoyed having a healthy baby. Again there were frequent references to being pregnant and feeling the baby move. References to the midwives were less frequent, but over one fifth of the Ashford and Deptford women said that what they had enjoyed most was their relationship with their particular midwife, while home births and antenatal home visits from the midwives also featured among the most enjoyable features of pregnancy and birth with some women.

The personal enjoyment of pregnancy and birth came through clearly in some of the interviews, as a Lewisham woman said: 'When you're pregnant it's almost like a dream world. Everyone's so wonderful. It's the attention you get. And seeing someone else who's pregnant in the street – you look at each other and smile. People treat you quite differently.'

A Deptford woman had had an equally good experience: 'At delivery the baby slid out. [The midwife] showed me the afterbirth and I touched it. It's a very spiritual thing. It put me in touch with my roots.' However, some people took a rather more functional view of the same thing, but with equally satisfactory results, it appeared, as an Ashford woman explained: 'The midwife dissected the afterbirth for my husband. He likes to know how things work. He was pleased about that.'

We asked the women whether their midwife had contributed to their positive memories of the pregnancy and birth. There were fairly marked differences among the areas. All but one of the Deptford women said that their midwife had contributed to their positive memories, a view shared by over 80 per cent of the Ashford women and just over three-quarters of the Lewisham women.

The main contributions made by the midwives were again their friendliness, cheerfulness, willingness to give information, advice and support, and their ability to instil confidence in the women. In Deptford there were also comments that the midwives helped the women to feel clever and confident and in control, which, interestingly, were seldom mentioned by women in other areas.

Some midwives clearly had particular skills, as a Deptford woman explained: 'I was very impressed by the way she allowed us to take control. She slipped into the background. She did it in such a way that we almost didn't notice. She took a back seat and let my husband hold the baby. She took photographs. She just kicked off her shoes and she was like a part of the family. I wish more mums could have that opportunity.'

Another Deptford woman also described a similar situation: 'She's very enthusiastic. She loves her job and it rubs off. It makes you feel it's a great thing having babies – that it's interesting and worthwhile. She became a friend really. It's like having a sister. She met the whole family.'

The familiarity and trust built up with the midwife during the antenatal period was clearly important to many women. An Ashford woman explained: 'We had seen her a lot during the pregnancy. There were lots of things to talk about – not just the birth – and it took my mind off things.' Another Ashford woman confirmed the need for trust: 'She was good during the delivery because she said, "Listen to me – push when I say and you'll have no stitches," and I pricked up my ears and did that – and she was right.'

And some women clearly still missed the contact they had established with their midwives, like another Ashford woman: 'At the end of the ten days afterwards when we said goodbye it was like losing a friend. We'd been through such a lot together.'

Negative memories of pregnancy and birth

But did the women have any negative memories of the pregnancy and birth? Given the strength of the positive memories it was perhaps surprising to find that over two-thirds of the Lewisham and Ashford women and nearly three-quarters of the Deptford women did.

What were the problems? They mainly centred on physical discomfort or pain. Of those with negative memories, well over half the Lewisham women, over one third in Ashford and over a quarter in Deptford mentioned physical problems during their pregnancy. Over a quarter of the Deptford women and one in six of the Lewisham women, but no-one in Ashford spoke of the pain in labour or delivery. This was perhaps related to the relatively low level of pain relief taken by the Deptford women.

Nearly a quarter of the Deptford women spoke of personal or family problems they had experienced during their pregnancy, although this was hardly mentioned in the other areas. Other negative memories included lack of information or poor care by the hospital staff, uncertainty about the type of delivery, long or difficult labours, postnatal pain, diagnosis of problems in pregnancy, cancelled or inadequate antenatal classes and lack of communication between midwives.

The physical discomfort or pain in pregnancy or labour were the aspects of the pregnancy and birth which were enjoyed least by the women. However, negative aspects of their midwifery care were mentioned by a small but vociferous minority of women, and these were by no means restricted only to the lack of communication between hospital staff and the midwifery group practice midwives which featured throughout these interviews.

Some of the lack of cooperation clearly amounted to lack of care, as an Ashford woman observed: 'The worst memory is that all I kept getting from the hospital was, "We shouldn't really be dealing with you because you're JACANES." For all they knew my baby could be dying inside me and you kept getting this stupid remark.'

Her experience was echoed both in Ashford and in Lewisham: 'The registrar was rude and patronising. She spoke to me as if I didn't have a brain. It seems to me there is a tension between the hospital staff and the midwives and you're caught in the middle.'

The apparent exclusiveness of the midwifery group practices could work the other way round as well, as a Deptford woman noted: 'It would have been nice to have a chance to see a consultant. They didn't say you could see one if you want. I didn't know until the end that I could have seen one. And they didn't say, "Are you sure you want the baby at home?" Doctors didn't feature. I went to see my GP out of courtesy.'

The lack of contact with GPs has also been a recurrent theme in this research, and again the Ashford woman who developed diabetes in pregnancy must be remembered: 'I felt so ill and I didn't know why. I felt so bad I went to see my GP and he tested my blood sugar and said, "My God!" He nearly had a heart attack.'

On the whole the women thought there was little that their named midwife could have done to alleviate their problems in pregnancy and childbirth, but some thought that more frequent attention to their physical needs, particularly in pain relief, could have helped, while others were rather uneasy about their care in general.

Relationships with the midwives

We asked the women whether their relationship with their named midwife had been satisfactory throughout. In Deptford all the women said that it had been, but a small number of women in other areas said that it had not. It should not be completely surprising that not all relationships of this kind are satisfactory and it is perhaps more surprising that so many relationships were so good.

The problems were usually very individual and mostly related to personal incompatibility, but in one or two cases related to lack of support postnatally in breastfeeding. Some women were able to change their midwife, but the system was not set up to facilitate this. One woman remarked: 'It would have been nice to choose your midwife.' Perhaps there is something to be learned here about offering choice in pregnancy and childbirth. It is not so simple as choosing the type of lead professional.

Comparison with previous midwifery care

We have seen that three-quarters of the Lewisham and Deptford women and nearly 60 per cent of the Ashford women interviewed after the birth of their babies had had previous maternities. We asked them whether they thought that the care that they had had from their midwives in this pregnancy was any different from the care they had had from midwives in previous pregnancies.

There were differences between the areas, but some of these related to the women being unable to make a judgement, while in other cases the women had had the same midwife in past pregnancies – one fifth of the Deptford women, for example, had had the same midwife before.

The Ashford women were the group most likely to have found a difference between the midwifery care on this occasion and on past occasions.

The comments mainly divided into positive comments about this pregnancy and adverse comments about previous pregnancies, and followed the pattern already established in these interviews. Women liked the time, the personal care, the continuity of carer, the greater flexibility of appointments and the involvement of family which they had highlighted as positive aspects of the care offered by the MGPs.

Their main criticisms of previous midwifery care related to seeing different people each time, seeing too many people, not knowing the midwife at the birth, long waits and lack of flexibility in appointments. One third of the Deptford women, but far fewer in the other areas, stressed that the midwifery care in their previous pregnancies had been too 'clinical'.

Again there were criticisms of previous hospital care, with references to feeling on a 'conveyor belt', rushed midwives who 'kept looking at their watches', tired midwives who 'wanted to be quick and break my waters', midwives who were 'always prodding and poking'. A Lewisham woman summarised the views of a number of women: 'I felt a nuisance when I asked questions last time, but this time I didn't. I felt I was just a slab of meat with the midwife last time. I think you get the worst treatment from the midwives in the hospital. I think they could improve on their attitude.'

Over one in ten of the women in Lewisham and Ashford mentioned that they had seen much more of their GPs in previous pregnancies, which some of them had found reassuring, as an Ashford woman explained: 'Last time you went to the surgery to see them and you saw them much more frequently. You were constantly monitored. So it did seem a bit strange not seeing your midwife so often. You got used to the doctor too. This time I went back to the GP for the six weeks postnatal check and she said, "You've had this baby and I didn't even know."'

But not everyone was so keen on shared care, and some of the Deptford women were vociferous in their criticism: 'With the DOMINO scheme there's a lot of chopping and changing and different faces. We didn't even have one of the six midwives that we'd met. We had someone from outside. And Deptford midwives have a lot more time. You don't feel that you're in a twenty minute slot.'

Satisfaction with midwifery group practice care

The women reported a high level of satisfaction with the care they received from the midwifery group practices. All the women using the Deptford MGP said that they were very satisfied with their overall experience, compared with 83 per cent in Lewisham and 88 per cent in Ashford. 13 per cent in Lewisham and 7 per cent in Ashford were fairly satisfied. 5 per cent in Lewisham and 2 per cent in Ashford were a bit dissatisfied, while 2 per cent in Ashford were very dissatisfied.

The two main reasons given for satisfaction with the midwifery group practices were the high professional standard of care given and the friendliness of the midwives. There were differences between the areas, with 50 per cent of the Deptford women mentioning the high professional standards of the midwives as a reason for their satisfaction, compared with a quarter of the women in the other two areas. On the other hand, nearly 50 per cent of the Ashford women stressed the friendliness of the midwives, compared with one third in Lewisham and one fifth in Deptford.

Other important factors in satisfaction were:

- being treated like a 'human being' or an individual (mentioned by a quarter of the women overall but most often in Lewisham)

- continuity of carer (mentioned by more than one fifth in Lewisham and Ashford but less often in Deptford)

- the reassurance offered by the midwives (mentioned by one third of the Ashford women, but fewer in the other areas)

- being able to call the midwife 'at any time' (mentioned by one fifth of the Deptford women and one in ten in the other areas).

Women mentioned a variety of other factors contributing to their satisfaction. Over one in ten in Lewisham liked the home antenatal visits, especially in the evenings; one fifth of the Deptford women liked being asked what they themselves wanted to do and being offered choices (hardly mentioned by other women); the involvement of the family; the opportunity to have a home birth; the time given at appointments; the convenience and the avoidance of hospital visits.

Some women liked everything about the midwives, and much could be learnt about good practice from their accounts, like that of a woman in Lewisham: 'They made me feel comfortable. I didn't know her that long and I would tell her things that I would not tell my doctors. I told her I had piles and I could not tell my doctor. She was always smiling even though she must have been often very tired.'

The continuity of care given by most midwives helped to engender trust, as an Ashford woman explained: 'It's just a positive thing to have the same midwife. They know you and you don't have to explain everything. It felt good not to be shunted from one health professional to another.'

And another Deptford woman highlighted another aspect of the care: 'We were treated first class. We don't have money. I'm black, street-wise – that was good. I'm not white, middle class, living in a nice big house. Equal opportunities – that's what I liked.'

But not everyone was very satisfied, and even among those who were there were still aspects of the care that some women found less satisfactory. The overwork of the Lewisham midwives was noted by several women: 'There were delays. It was 15 minutes before the baby was cleaned. Then it was half an hour before I was stitched. I had my legs up in the air while I waited to be stitched. I don't want to remember this because it still gives me nightmares. I felt that this happened because I was only assigned to one midwife on the project.'

A Deptford woman was also a bit dubious about her care: 'The only thing – if I'd been in hospital the tear might not have been so bad and I might not have needed stitching. They could have done a quick snip. The doctor who came to do the stitches showed them what they could have done.'

The assumption that women do not want to see their GPs was marked among some of the midwives, but it appeared that some women felt uneasy about not being offered choices, as a Lewisham woman explained: 'I saw the same midwife all the way through this time, where before I saw the midwife and the doctor. I'd have preferred shared care. I'd rather have seen my doctor. I saw him for a query with the baby's heartbeat but that wasn't a proper antenatal. I'd have had more confidence in our doctor.'

Some of the Deptford women clearly felt that they were drawn into an unfortunate tension between the midwives and their own GPs: 'They're not really fully integrated into the medical system, and communications can break down with hospitals and GPs and so on. When you go to your GP about something they're very suspicious of the practice.'

The position of the Deptford midwives was a cause for concern for some women: 'My only criticism is that what they offer is not mainstream in the NHS. They are regarded as radical. They are very intelligent and it's a vocation, not a job, and they question everything and they encourage you to question. The hospital midwives just go through the rules and regulations and that is very conservative. I think hospital midwifery is shoddy compared to what these midwives are offering.'

And there were indications that the closeness of the relationship with the midwife had sometimes engendered a level of dependency which was going to be hard for the women to relinquish. A Deptford woman said – 'I just wished she'd lived here with me for the nine months, that's all' – and her sentiments were echoed in Ashford – 'I didn't like the times when she couldn't come. I would have liked her all the time.'

On the other hand, as we have seen, some Ashford women were concerned about the infrequency of the antenatal consultations with midwives. Some felt a need for more information: 'I wonder if they could see the first time mums more often. And I think it would be better if they wrote down in their notes what they were going to talk about next time, because a couple of times she forgot and didn't cover the things she said she would.' Her views were shared by another Ashford woman: 'I felt everything I wanted to ask was such a silly thing and I'd not bother them. I got most of the information I needed out of books.'

And another clearly needed more help: 'I am a single mum on my own. I could have had counselling. Being pregnant was very emotional anyway. I was very upset about the father – he abandoned me. Someone should try and see – "Does this lady need someone to talk to?" I think that might have been good for me.'

We have already seen that liaison between midwives and health visitors appeared rather haphazard, and a number of women pointed up problems: 'I wish there was more cross-over to include the health visitor side so you wouldn't have this contradiction in advice. It would be nice not to be confronted by this new person on your doorstep who doesn't know you from Adam.'

Assessment

We have seen so often in this research that many of the positive aspects of the midwifery care offered by the midwifery group practices highlighted practice in hospitals which was less than adequate. Perhaps one of the main messages from this evaluation is that hospital practice should be improved before it is assumed that midwifery group practices are the only way of running midwifery care.

An Ashford woman gave a graphic account: 'I only went to the hospital once and that was to see (the consultant). It was like a cattle market up there. I had seen four people in the space of half an hour. One person weighed me, one person took my blood pressure, one checked my urine and then I saw the consultant. I came out and said to my husband, "Thank God I don't have to do this all the way through."'

The high standard of care offered and the trust engendered in many of the relationships with the midwives may well serve as a model for how health services of all types should be delivered. A Deptford woman said: 'I only wish I could get a guarantee to have the same care if I had another baby. I was more satisfied than with almost any other aspect of my life.'

Her views were repeated in each area by many women. Much could be learnt from the accounts from women reported in the last two chapters, not only about good midwifery practice but also about good health care in general. Some of the care, time and personal attention offered by the midwifery group practices to women who were not sick might seem to be of an intensity that was not always appropriate, but there were many clear messages in these accounts regarding good practice which could easily be incorporated into mainstream practice by less dedicated practitioners with less time and resources available.

Chapter 7

The midwifery group practice midwives

All group practice midwives who were in post at the beginning of the monitoring period were interviewed during May and June 1994 to establish a benchmark for their aims and expectations and to identify the criteria they themselves would use for measuring their achievements. On a similar basis we also interviewed the senior midwifery manager in two of the midwifery group practices (MGPs), but not in Deptford where the group was self-managing.

The midwives and their managers were interviewed again at the end of the monitoring period to reflect on their experiences of working in an MGP, to comment on characteristic features of this model of service provision and to assess whether or not the model they had developed could be transferred to other areas in its present form. The timing of the final interviews took account of staff changes during the monitoring period, with the three midwives who left the Deptford MGP being interviewed before moving on in the spring of 1995. The final round of interviews also included the practice manager at Deptford, who joined the project part way through, and the health resource worker whose responsibilities at the start of the project had also included practice management.

In reporting on these interviews we show that while some key differences between the three MGPs emerged, there were also a number of common themes which have significance for the replication and sustainability of this model of care provision.

Setting up the midwifery group practices

Recruitment and selection
The process of recruitment and selection was different for individual midwives, both between and within the three MGPs. The biggest differences were, however, between Lewisham and Ashford on the one hand, and Deptford on the other.

Lewisham and Ashford

In Lewisham and Ashford (JACANES) some of the MGP midwives were involved at the start in putting together the bids and assembling the teams. As one midwife in Ashford explained: 'In June last year three of us formed a small group. Then there was the Cumberlege Report and a request for pilot schemes to be submitted. We were already trying to work out a system to form a midwifery group. Then the applications were asked for quite soon after that.'

It was generally felt that while some of the preparatory thinking had already been done, insufficient planning time had been available. In the words of one midwife: 'We had to formulate who would be on the team. Time was very short and no planning had been done. We knew from other people's writing that successful teams were planned for a year or even two. Less successful teams weren't planned so well.'

The small core of midwives in Lewisham and Ashford who were involved in developing their respective bids were joined by other midwives who responded to job advertisements. A point made strongly by a number of midwives in both MGPs was that they did not choose whom they worked with and for some this was seen as a potential weakness.

Another important recruitment issue was the balance required between community and hospital midwives. As one Lewisham midwife commented: 'There were problems. Those who presented first were community based. In between the bids and internal adverts we were told it could only be three hospital and three community midwives so it did not deplete the service.'

Deptford

The setting up process was quite different in Deptford where a core group of previously independent midwives came together to form the MGP. They were joined by other midwives who were known to them, and who were attracted by their philosophy of working. As one of the founding members explained: 'Ever since I've worked independently I've worked with a colleague and was in touch with other professional midwives. We were all good friends and we worked together with the same philosophy. We gradually talked of forming a group practice. We were all, in effect, private with payment from women, although we've done a lot of "Robin Hooding". We all shared a dream of one day being able to work in this way but being funded by the NHS. I didn't only want to work for rich people. Last year there was the Winterton report and then the Cumberlege Report. She actually took evidence from us. South East Thames decided to fund two projects and invited bids and we saw ourselves being involved. We knew we were on course.'

Skills brought to the job

In all three MGPs few of the midwives felt that they had brought skills to the group that were not offered by others in the MGP. Most highlighted their general commitment and enthusiasm, while individual midwives referred to specific experience in, for example, midwifery education; parentcraft skills; epidural top-ups; and suturing. In some activities individual midwives took the lead where they and other group members felt they had particular experience: for example, in producing a document on standards of care, or in offering the option of a waterbirth.

Aims of the MGP pilot projects as set up by SETRHA

At both the beginning and end of the monitoring period midwives reflected on South East Thames Regional Health Authority's (SETRHA) main aims in setting up MGP pilot projects. SETRHA's aims were primarily seen to focus on specific service objectives, with the overriding goals of achieving more satisfaction both for the women using the service and for midwives. For example, '...to provide continuity of care and carer, choice and control for the client, and job satisfaction for the midwife.' For another midwife these objectives stemmed from a particular view of pregnancy: 'Their overall aim is that they appreciate that pregnancy and birth is not an illness and they want to give women the opportunity to participate in the decision making element of their pregnancy – giving choice and therefore control.'

The MGPs were also seen as a means for SETRHA to assess the benefits and costs of implementing the model of care promoted by *Changing Childbirth*. In the words of one midwifery manager it was important, '...to establish a model that could be replicated. To establish a firm foundation for *Changing Childbirth* – properly evaluated.'

While not wanting to detract from the value of the pilot projects one or two midwives at the outset admitted to being unsure of SETRHA's specific aims. At the end of the study a concern emerged that the people involved in setting up the projects at SETRHA had left and that as time went on the original aims became less clear.

Aims of the individual midwifery group practices

Not surprisingly the aims of the individual MGPs mirrored, in most respects, those laid down by SETRHA. Indeed, one of the Deptford midwives felt that not only were the aims of their practice in line with SETRHA's aims but that, 'I think we informed them in the first place. It is circular. They haven't put up anything we wouldn't have advocated in the first place. Historically a lot of the ideas came from us.'

Some differences in structure and practice were noted, however, in both Ashford and Deptford. Two of the Ashford midwives commented at the outset that their caseload was larger than SETRHA envisaged. One explained that this was due to the fact that 'we also look after the mums booked for hospital delivery under consultant care', in addition to looking after the 'uncomplicated' women. A distinction was drawn between the type of care they were able to provide in each case: 'Those that are complicated are delivered by the hospital staff. The continuity of care is for the uncomplicated. We have a caseload of 550 and it would be impossible for six of us to handle all of those deliveries.' As noted elsewhere, action was taken during the course of the monitoring period to reduce the caseload size by focusing the work of JACANES on the 'uncomplicated' women and setting up a second MGP (JACANES II) to provide midwifery care to the 'complicated' cases.

Several of the Deptford midwives highlighted ways in which their practice differed not just from the aims laid down by SETRHA but also from the other two MGPs. Deptford MGP had its own premises and was not attached to any GP practices. It operated on the basis of self referral and direct access to the midwives. The practice was formed as a partnership and was self-managing. Referring to the recommendations of *Changing Childbirth,* one of the Deptford midwives also commented that they aimed to achieve higher targets and in a shorter time period than envisaged in that report.

In drawing to our attention how much group discussion there had been about the aims of their MGPs, many of the midwives remarked that the MGP environment had been more open and conducive to discussion about aims and practice than any other working environment they had previously experienced. As one of the Ashford midwives explained: 'We meet weekly and one of these meetings each month includes our midwifery manager. Because it's a pilot we're changing our specifications fairly regularly to adjust to the needs. Also we can talk fairly frankly. I've not been in many environments before where we've been able to.' The benefit of frank discussion was also emphasised by the senior midwifery manager.

Similarly in Deptford when the midwives initially came together to form the MGP there was much enthusiasm for discussing aims: 'We discuss it [aims] all the time. I can't underplay how much discussion we have. It has been really wonderful having a practice base where we can meet and discuss things and being in a community centre with other health based projects is very exciting.'

Over the monitoring period the nature of the team meetings tended to change for all the MGPs as they became established, with discussion becoming more reflective and focusing on current work, rather than aims and set-up issues. Looking to the future, however, became an issue for all three groups, with one of the Lewisham midwives explaining: 'We can't make plans any more because no-one will tell us what is happening to the MGP.' For Deptford in particular the difficulties in securing funding soon had an impact on the nature of what was discussed at group meetings: 'We are always discussing project aims – how to access target groups and so on, but we have a clear idea of what the practice is about. Recently the situation has become more political. How can we convince the Commission that we are doing the right thing?'

Access

Midwives were conscious that the route of access to midwifery services was different between the three MGPs. We were reminded that women were referred to the Lewisham and Ashford MGPs through the GP surgeries which were participating in the pilot project. As one Lewisham midwife observed: 'These GPs were identified as supplying the number of women we could handle. We meet women at classes who would like to be part of the practice but we don't want to be seen as poaching. We'd be inundated.' Additionally, where ex-community midwives were concerned a few referrals came from past clients. As one such midwife observed: 'It's very difficult to refuse someone you've delivered twice before.'

While midwives saw the benefits attached to working from GP surgeries, this also made it difficult for the midwives to be the first point of access. One Lewisham midwife commented that access was through GPs because: 'That's what the GPs wanted. And because we haven't got accommodation anywhere else it might be best now. I hope we become the first point of contact. For that we need a visible place in the community. Our biggest problem is we're homeless.'

This was not a problem for the Deptford midwives who had a permanent and visible base in a local community centre. The majority of their referrals were self referrals who had either been past clients of the independent midwives, or had learned about the practice by word of mouth or through using the pregnancy testing service. Some had also become more aware of the services offered by the Deptford MGP through attending the antenatal classes run for all-comers by the midwives, or by seeing the shop front. Few referrals were from GPs and other professionals. In the words of one of the midwives: 'Women find out we're based around the corner or know someone who has been cared for by one of us in the past. We also hope to go into the community for women who aren't on the grapevine and to offer free pregnancy testing. In the long term perhaps GPs could offer it as an option but I think that's quite a long way off.'

Publicity

There was some concern in the Lewisham and Ashford MGPs that '...women don't know they don't have to go through a doctor.' An Ashford midwife felt that this was partly because the service was not publicised. They had been asked by their managers not to publicise the service because this would risk giving the impression of 'superior' and 'inferior' services. There was also the more practical reason highlighted by a Lewisham midwife: 'I'd love to publicise it but at the moment it is not fair because of the way our women are being recruited from three group practices. We couldn't take any more.' In fact, over time it emerged that some women were changing their GPs in order to get access to the Lewisham MGP and this was seen as a contributory factor to their high caseload.

In Deptford publicity was seen as vital in order to attract clients given that there was no automatic referral route through GPs. Nevertheless during the monitoring period midwives had mixed feelings about the extent to which the service should be publicised, in view of the uncertainty about their continued funding and the constraints this placed on booking clients whose pregnancy would go beyond the guaranteed funding period.

Nature of the caseload

Midwives in the Lewisham and Ashford MGPs thought that there were no distinct differences between the women using their services and those using other local midwifery services. This was largely because the majority of the women were referred from the participating GP practices. Nevertheless, there was a general feeling in both MGPs that there were particular groups of women that they were able to help. In Lewisham it was mentioned that the MGP provided more choice for high risk women, for women having their first babies and for women with a fear of hospitals. In Ashford the model of care was seen as particularly appropriate for women who were poor users of mainstream services. Illustrating this point one of the midwives told us: 'I do two surgeries. One has a lot of social class IV and V women who under the old system would have been non-attenders at the hospital. With community care there is less need to chase them. It has improved their outcomes.'

At the start of the monitoring period there was a general feeling among the Deptford midwives that their case-load composition was in a transitionary phase. Most of their clients were self-referrals and early on many had previously been clients of the independent midwives who had formed the MGP. These clients, according to one of the midwives, were '...more aware people who read more, people who think more about what they want. Women who are more assertive and able to fight their own battles.' Increasingly the Deptford midwives aimed to boost the number of bookings with women in the target groups which were specified in their contract with purchasers. Reflecting at the end of the study on particular groups of women which the MGP had been able to help these midwives referred to '...women in the target groups – particularly the community from Vietnam. Those with pregnancy bereavement, and teenagers. Also those in the mental health category. A lot of women whose lives are on the edge'

Views on existing service provision

A view was prevalent across all three MGPs that needs were not being met by existing services. Lack of continuity of care and carer was seen as a particular problem. An Ashford midwife explained: 'Other community midwives don't deliver babies. They don't give continuity of care. Some community midwives don't want to be contacted or spend too much time.' A similar point was made in Deptford: 'Sometimes women find it difficult to get hold of a midwife to talk to. They rarely see the same one again and keep on having to repeat the story.'

Lack of choice for women about who would provide their care and about type and place of birth was also identified across the MGPs as a major issue, as was the unpredictability of the standard of care received. A graphic description of the problem was provided by an Ashford midwife: 'Within this area there are women who are not being offered a choice of carer. They don't even know that it should be offered. There are individual midwives who are not keeping up their practices or skills in the labour wards and are not prepared to work unsociable hours.' Similarly in Deptford: 'I've come across many women who have wanted continuity of carer or a home birth and have not been able to book these. And in antenatal preparation and support in pregnancy. Women seem to have very traumatic experiences at birth with no one to talk to about it afterwards.'

There was considerable support for the view that there were insufficient community midwifery staff and that this affected the standard and type of care that women currently received. For one of the Deptford midwives this was part of a bigger problem that current services were configured to meet the organisation's needs and not the needs of women: 'They [current services] are a disaster. Nationally, not just this region. Because the whole maternity structure now serves the structure rather than the women. Too much resource goes into the infrastructure – the running of the institution and the needs of professionals and workers within it. In practical terms it means women have to fit in to what suits the institution.'

Comparison with existing service provision

Not surprisingly, at the end of the study period virtually all of the MGP midwives felt that their group practice had improved the services available locally and offered women something that they could not get elsewhere. This was often attributed to the way the service was organised, and not because they saw themselves as better midwives. In comparing their own approach with existing services the midwives in all three MGPs emphasised that continuity of care and carer were much improved. They also pointed to increased choice of lead professional, and of type and place of delivery, as this Ashford midwife noted: 'We give the mums a choice as to who they want as their lead professional, type and place of delivery and format of their antenatal care. Plus we have a fall-back system – if one is not available she will know the replacement midwife already.'

Midwives in Lewisham and Deptford in particular felt they had more flexibility which made them more responsive to user needs. In Deptford this was coupled with a feeling that midwives were more directly accessible than elsewhere and had more control over the way they worked: 'It's about midwives doing the job that they are trained for rather than being an obstetric handmaiden.' Interlinked with midwifery care the Deptford MGP also offered women a shopfront service which operated as a 'women's health resource'. The manager of this service explained: *'Changing Childbirth* is all about reaching women and especially the local community. It is also about information. The woman's health service offers all sorts of things. This is how the practice has responded to *Changing Childbirth.'*

Comparison with previous work experience

In drawing a comparison between the services offered by their MGP and other midwifery services the midwives often referred to their own previous experiences in midwifery. Many of the differences mentioned echoed midwives' comments about more continuity, choice and flexibility afforded by the MGPs.

Several of the midwives said that they felt more in control in their current job because they now had a known caseload and the support of their colleagues in the MGP. This was the experience of the Deptford midwife who said: 'I find the on-call I do now much easier to cope with than I did before. I think that it's because of the caseload. I know when the phone rings who is likely to have gone into labour and what is likely to happen. I find this type of on-call much less stressful than on-call where any number of women you've never met could ring in.' Another important difference identified was the opportunity, provided by greater continuity of care and carer, to build up a deeper relationship with the women using their services.

A number of the midwives in each of the MGPs felt that they were involved in more management and administration than they were used to and while some found this a chore, others, like an Ashford midwife, viewed it more positively: 'I'm currently doing the duty rota and that is a new kind of administration which I find interesting. It's quite a challenge.'

Midwives who had come to the MGP from a hospital post were more likely to highlight differences associated with the fact that the MGPs were community based. These differences included a closer working relationship with GPs.

Importantly for job satisfaction, several of the midwives pointed out that they were able to make fuller use of their skills in the MGPs. Greater autonomy also brings greater responsibility and, as emphasised by one of the Lewisham midwives, the need to be clinically sharper: 'Because I have overall responsibility for them I have to look into all aspects of their care because there is no likelihood of anyone else picking it up if you missed it.'

Specific features of the MGPs' approach

Midwives talked in more depth about their understanding of 'midwife-led care' and about how they had tried to ensure that choice and continuity of care were achieved in practice.

Midwife-led care

Different definitions of 'midwife-led care' were apparent both within and between the three MGPs, but a central thread in all of these was the role of the midwife as main carer. For example: 'In the old system people booked under the consultant. Now the midwife is the main carer, the person the mum is booked under.'

A number of the midwives were keen to ensure that the definition highlighted the partnership between the midwife and the woman. A Lewisham midwife defined 'midwife-led care' as occurring: 'Where the midwife is in control in partnership with the woman throughout. She will make referrals where necessary, but concentrates on the pregnancy rather than her illnesses or medicalisation.'

It should be recognised that some of the midwives found 'midwife-led care' an ambiguous term. Frequently definitions drew on the concept of the 'lead professional' with the midwife acting as '...the lead professional, looking after the mother through the whole episode of care, bringing in other help if complications arise or if the mother wishes.' However, this association did not necessarily add clarity because there was also confusion over the concept of 'lead professional' as this observation from a Lewisham midwife illustrated: 'The midwife is the lead professional. The only other thing is the consultant. That's one of the ambiguous questions. To me the midwife is the one constant person in the whole thing. If a woman is going to have a caesarean why is the consultant the lead professional? She is still under our care, even if the consultant tells us when he wants her to come in. I've met other girls on this pilot and they have the same question. Who is the lead professional? Another example is a woman who is booked at home under her GP. Does that make the GP the lead professional? Again, I don't know.'

This ambiguity was also emphasised among the Deptford midwives: 'We as a group are about to have a meeting to thrash this out. The person who gives the majority of care is the lead professional – normally the midwives. Cumberlege hasn't helped. *Changing Childbirth* talks about lead professionals. I don't feel I'm any less accountable than a consultant with women of high risk because I'm out there.'

Choice of carer

Midwives in Lewisham and Ashford said that the majority of women who used their MGPs would at some stage be offered the choice of midwife, GP or obstetrician-led care. In most cases the choice was offered by the midwife at the initial booking visit, but for some women the range of options might have been discussed earlier when they visited their GP.

In Deptford the issue was raised that some women had already exercised their choice in opting to book with the MGP, and this applied particularly to late bookers. The extent of discussion about alternative options was likely to be more tailored to the particular client but midwives said that clients were made aware of what was available: 'At booking we tell them what is on offer. We talk about home birth and DOMINO and antenatal care. We say they can book all their care with us. They can have all with a GP. They can go to the hospital and see midwives in the antenatal clinic. I don't put it in terms of lead professional to women because if I don't understand what it is how can they?'

The midwives in Lewisham and Ashford said that if a woman opted for GP-led care they nearly always continued to provide midwifery care within the midwifery group practice. In Deptford this was less common. One of the midwives explained that she would only work in this way if there was a medical or obstetric reason: 'Otherwise there is no point in booking with us. We're not planning to do GP shared care. We'll do it but it's messy because she will not see us that much. And it's only really shared care if GPs will come to the birth. Only two in this area will.'

Midwives in all three MGPs continued to provide midwifery care to women who needed to be referred to a consultant obstetrician at some point in their pregnancy, but this gave rise to some confusion about who was then the lead professional. It was pointed out that the consultant might provide the specialist element but that the midwife was still likely to see the woman most often and to be the one who coordinated her care. In most cases the MGP midwife would also go with the woman to see the consultant. The Deptford midwives in particular felt: 'It comes down to being unclear what lead professional means.' This lack of clarity was more than a definitional problem because it has implications for accountability which we discuss in Chapter 10.

Continuity of care

We asked the midwives what steps each MGP had taken to ensure better continuity of care for women than that provided by existing services. Midwives in all three MGPs highlighted the fact that they had their own caseloads and that the women in turn had a named midwife: 'We have personalised caseloads – we look after the women we book all the way through. If we involve other health professionals, we will go with them to appointments, providing the continuity.' Midwives were not allocated women where the expected delivery date (EDD) was around the time of their annual leave.

Midwives in all the MGPs also stressed the importance of ensuring that the women met more than one midwife during their antenatal care, thus ensuring continuity of care if not individual carer. For example, an Ashford midwife explained: 'We have a "drop in" session where any of the mums can come along and meet all six midwives.' We were also told of simple things: 'A photograph of the group helps. It's nice to know who is coming to see you.' In Deptford the midwives emphasised the use of primary and secondary midwives or pairing: 'Continuity of care is guaranteed except in the case of unexpected sickness. The primary midwife does almost all care. The secondary does back-up care.'

The on-call system, mobile telephones and bleeps were seen as important mechanisms in ensuring continuity, as were flexible working hours and home visits: 'We have mobile phones and the clients can contact us at any time when we're on-call. And we go to see them at home rather than a hospital. You are mobile; you can be here and there; you are not in a fixed environment.' Regular contact and meetings between midwives to discuss and review caseloads were also seen as important in supporting continuity.

In all three MGPs the motivation of midwives and their commitment to shared goals were cited as overriding strengths in achieving greater continuity of care. In the words of a Deptford midwife: 'We have a common philosophy. Women have access to all of us through the groups. If a woman has to have other than the midwife she is booked with she can be sure she will not get someone with a different approach. They are booked with the practice, not just the first and second midwife. I feel confident in them getting any of us.' Similarly one of the Ashford midwives confirmed: 'We work very much as a team. Women do get continuity. We all have one aim and goal. I'm not putting other midwives down, but even under team care it is pot luck who would deliver them. I have full confidence that what I've promised other midwives will facilitate.'

At the end of the study around half of the midwives confirmed that they had experienced some difficulties in providing continuity of care and carer for women, with this being more of a problem in Lewisham than in Ashford and Deptford. Difficulties that had been encountered were mostly to do with the logistics of providing cover for holidays or sick leave, or with the unpredictable timing or length of labour. In Ashford, and to a lesser extent Lewisham, a high caseload was also seen as a weakness in trying to achieve continuity.

Tiredness was a crucial factor which could made continuity difficult, as an Ashford midwife indicated: 'If we've been up all night you might have to get somebody else to cover you. We were getting too tired. We were too ambitious. We took it literally – 24 hour cover.' A colleague of hers added: 'We try to overdo it sometimes. We are perhaps too committed to the women and the project and want to make it work. This goes back to flexibility and could be a weakness for the future. Could you expect this from all midwives? I think not.' It is clear that some of the midwives had too high expectations of themselves. In the words of one midwifery manager, these were fuelled by 'uninformed optimism'. Her concern was whether these expectations could be sustained when 'realistic pessimism' set in.

In discussing the implications of these difficulties in the end of study interviews it was common for midwives themselves to reflect on the feasibility of continuity and to draw a distinction between continuity of care and continuity of carer. Whereas at the start of the study they tended to emphasise the ideal of the named midwife providing all or most of a woman's care, in the light of experience they were more inclined to guarantee that a woman would receive care from a known midwife in the MGP, rather than one-to-one care with the named midwife.

This view was put forcibly by a midwife in the Lewisham practice: 'I'm not sure that all the midwives understand totally what a group practice is. I've delivered some I don't know. We should be a group of seven midwives delivering care to women. We began being retentive of our women. It changed over time. I never say I will deliver your baby – rather the group practice will. I don't think it has to be the same midwife. We need to stop feeling guilty.' The same midwife argued: 'Continuity of care can be achieved without continuity of carer. Continuity of carer does not mean good quality care. That's not the end of it. It has to be something deeper.'

The MGPs also demonstrate that continuity of carer can carry the risk of creating too a great a dependency in the relationship. This was recognised early on in the monitoring period by the Lewisham midwife who said: 'We do much more antenatal care at home and already I can see that we're building up a much deeper relationship with the mums from the beginning. We do the bookings, give them a contact number which is their lifeline. They're treating us like social workers or psychologists. We hear everything. I don't know if that is a good thing. If you've got 20 people on your books with all these problems there is only a certain amount you can carry with you. If they become very dependent on us it's very hard on them as well. This did not happen before unless there happened to be someone you saw regularly.'

The issue of dependency and its implications was raised across all three MGPs during the final interviews. We were told in Lewisham: 'Because it's one-to-one care if the relationship breaks down there is a problem. It's so close. If I don't like them and they don't like me there is a problem with communication. And if the midwife is sick the other midwives have to do a lot of work. If the mum is so involved with the midwife and the midwife can't see them it upsets the woman who doesn't like it at all. Put simply, if you have a very dependent woman and the midwife cannot provide care, the woman feels very let down.'

Choice of type and place of birth

Offering women a greater choice in terms of type and place of birth was also an objective of the MGPs and we asked midwives at what stage in their pregnancy women would normally make the decision between a home or hospital birth. In both Lewisham and Ashford women were most likely to make this decision at booking, particularly if they wanted a home birth, although some left it until midway or even later in their pregnancy. In contrast, all the Deptford midwives said that they were very flexible about it and women could make this decision, 'at any stage'.

All the midwives indicated that they spent a considerable amount of time with the women discussing the various options. As one Lewisham midwife emphasised, this discussion needed to be handled sensitively: 'You give her the advantages and disadvantages. You give her the choices. It's sometimes very difficult. You've got to be very neutral. The choice is up to her. If you are too subjective you can influence quite easily.' Midwives were likely to refer women to research findings and other written information if this was appropriate.

While most of the midwives had some previous experience of offering women a choice between home and hospital birth, six of the midwives had concerns at the start of the pilot about becoming involved in more home births. For some their concerns centred around lack of experience in home deliveries. In the previous 12 months (up until 1 April 1994) seven of the midwives (3 in Lewisham, 3 in Ashford and 1 in Deptford) had not actually supervised any home births. All but one of these, who was an ex-community midwife, had previously worked as hospital midwives immediately before joining one of the MGPs.

Others were worried about the actual or potential lack of support or back-up from GPs. One Ashford midwife said: 'I've had my hands rapped already. I was sent for. The GPs said they didn't want home deliveries. I said I couldn't refuse. They wanted me to tell the mums that they couldn't have a home delivery. I was told that the GPs would dissuade the mums. I've had an official letter saying I'm not to book home deliveries. But I'm booking my home deliveries and getting another GP to cover me. Home deliveries are taboo in the practice I'm in now.' A similar point was made by one of her colleagues: 'With some women who choose a home birth who are not totally suitable you may not have any medical back-up if the GP refuses to give care. It hasn't happened yet but the potential is there.'

At the end of the monitoring period we asked the midwives whether in working in the MGP they had in practice increased the extent to which they had offered women a choice between home and hospital births. Most of the midwives in Lewisham felt that they had, and that this had brought about an increase in the number of women opting for home births and had opened up home births to a wider range of people. It had also increased their own confidence in their skills, particularly where their previous experience was mostly hospital based: 'Clinically, all my experience was based in hospital. I wondered how I would cope and now I've done quite a few and it has built up my confidence and I've learned to improvise, to trust my own judgement. Sometimes it can be quite frightening, mostly because they trust you. If I say something, they want me to make the decision. It can be quite frightening, but you learn.'

In Ashford fewer midwives felt that their practice in offering choice over place of birth had changed, with several saying that they had previously offered the choice between home or hospital. Others indicated, however, that their involvement in births (both hospital and home deliveries) was more fulfilling since working with the MGP. As one described it: 'It is more like delivering a friend. When I was on the labour ward you had to start from scratch and it's hard to judge someone's capacity for pain.'

The Deptford midwives did not consider that they had increased the extent to which they offered a choice between home and hospital births whilst operating in the pilot, nor had the number of women opting for a home birth increased. Indeed, one of the midwives, who had previously operated in the area as an independent midwife, said for her personally: 'There has been a decrease because the women used to seek us out for home births. My home birth rate has dropped considerably. This was a worry. How would I keep birth 'normal' in hospital with all the intrusions on a physiological level. In spite of this the home birth rate [for the MGP] has stayed high. Few have opted for hospital.' Those midwives who had previously been independent found themselves becoming more involved in births in hospitals. They also welcomed the opportunity of opening up home births to people who would never before have been offered this option, for example, teenage girls.

In all projects it was pointed out that any increase in home births was not simply a result of the midwives offering choice, but was also due to a grapevine effect within the local communities. As one midwife explained: 'They did not know they had the choice before. They just thought they had to have a hospital birth. It's not just us. Now the scheme has been going for a while they talk to one another. They arrive knowing what they want. They hear from their friends. Word spreads.'

By the end of the monitoring period situations where a woman had opted for a home birth, when in the midwife's opinion a hospital birth would have been more appropriate, had occurred for ten of the midwives (5 in Lewisham, 4 in Ashford and 1 in Deptford). The outcomes they described varied considerably. In some instances the women had switched to hospital deliveries once the risks had been explained. In several instances the women had delivered at home and there had been no complications, but in two cases involving home births it was reported that the emergency services had been required. One of the midwives observed that she had learned a lot about estimating risk from exposure to these types of cases.

There were also instances where midwives (2 in Lewisham, 4 in Ashford and 6 in Deptford) had to deal with women opting for a home birth against the advice and wishes of their GP. In most of these cases the midwives reported that women had achieved a home delivery, but for some women a hospital delivery became necessary because of complications. Lewisham midwives said that the reasons for GPs advising against a home delivery were either that a home birth was considered unsafe because of obstetric complications, or because the GP was in principle against home births.

In Ashford a number of GPs were also said to be in principle against home births. One midwife explained: 'In my health centre GPs are against home deliveries. If she insists, they withdraw intrapartum back-up. We have no GP back-up.' They also felt that some GPs refused to become involved in home births because they did not have the necessary up-to-date skills.

The reasons given by Deptford midwives for GPs advising women against home births were broadly similar to those cited by Lewisham and Ashford but also demonstrated concern among GPs about home births for first babies and in cases of increased maternal age. The midwives were also aware of GPs' concerns about safety: 'A lot of GPs trained during the era when they were told home births were more dangerous. Research included all risks in home birth statistics. GPs are scared. They haven't caught up with the evidence. They hold on to the bio-medical perspective that it might be unsafe.'

Attractions of the job

At the beginning of the study midwives talked to us about what had attracted them to working with a group practice and the aspects they were particularly looking forward to. Providing continuity of care was emphasised by the Lewisham and Ashford midwives. As one explained: 'Over the years women have said to me so often how much they appreciate continuity of care. Sometimes they say, "Right at the end it wouldn't have mattered because I was in so much pain I didn't care," but for most of the time, for most women, that is what they want – to know the midwife who will be with them during labour.'

Flexibility of working and more autonomy in working and building up a relationship with the women were also anticipated. As one Lewisham midwife put it: 'Being able to actually work with the women without interference from the doctors. I saw it as an opportunity. And I was disillusioned with the way we were practising midwifery in the hospital. It was really difficult. You'd love to talk to the women and you couldn't make the time. You had other priorities and it was difficult and frustrating. With the training you've been given you want to be using it rather than being led.' Similar sentiments were expressed by the Ashford midwife who liked '...the increased responsibility and being able to give the choices - my hands aren't tied.'

The concept of a group practice and working in a supportive network of midwives had been attractive to many of the midwives. Associated with this was increased confidence in being able to hand over to colleagues in the MGP and know that the woman would receive a similar service, with no unnecessary interventions. In the words of an Ashford midwife: 'The fact of being able to go off duty and know another midwife [in the group] will care for your mother in the way they want. We are all different but we share the same philosophy.'

Reservations about the job

The majority of the midwives in all three practices admitted to having some reservations when they joined the MGPs. At the beginning of the monitoring period some highlighted the terms and conditions of the job, particularly the longer hours entailed by more deliveries and the amount of time on call. This was linked to concerns about exhaustion, burn-out and the impact of the job on family and social life. A Lewisham midwife described her concerns in this way: 'The demands on our own lives and on one's own partner or relationships. I still have reservations because I don't know that it is the only way of working to give most satisfaction to women and midwives. If midwives burn out you don't get good value care. I have reservations about it being seen as politically correct to work in this way.'

In one or two cases concerns about tiredness, particularly the longer hours entailed in more deliveries, were linked to anxieties about ensuring safe practice. An Ashford midwife commented that she was not anxious about the work itself, '...but the being on call and not knowing when I'm too tired and must hand over. You have a sense of desertion and failure even though it's not your fault that things are not normal'. This concern was shared by her colleague who was also anxious about '...being up all night sometimes when you're tired. You get to the stage when you have to ask if you are safe. You have to know when to call somebody else in to take over'.

Group relationships were another focus of concern for some midwives. Referring back to selection procedures, one Lewisham midwife said: 'We were told only "x" number of community midwives on the scheme so a lot of people held back from applying... We felt it was important to work with people who shared our philosophy of care but that didn't happen, and that was a huge worry. It wasn't a hospital/community thing, it was different ways of working.'

A colleague shared her concern: 'My main concern is that we should have chosen to work together. The job is very stressful and it's more than a job. It's to do with your life and you wouldn't choose to live with someone you didn't like. Communication may be a barrier or a challenge but it's still difficult. This is likely to continue to be a difficulty but I hope it's getting better.'

Even where self-selection had operated there was still some anxiety, as one of the Deptford midwives illustrated: 'I wondered if we would get on well. We're all very individualistic and powerful women. We've been very careful about not back-chatting and not talking about each other. There's one midwife I couldn't work with, but I don't have to.'

In all the MGPs there were some midwives who were worried about not fitting in with the group. One was concerned about '...not being good enough – could I keep up the standard? I'd got too hospitalised and would this show?' Another was aware that she needed 'people to be as motivated as me, especially in labour care', and that she had to learn patience and to allow other people to do what they wanted.

Some midwives were anxious about the extent to which they would be accepted by local GPs and consultant obstetricians: 'Would they accept midwife autonomy? Would they be able to lay off and not see us as working against them but attempting to cooperate for the betterment of the women?'

Job satisfaction

In the end of study interviews midwives echoed many of their earlier expectations in reflecting on the dimensions of job satisfaction obtained in working in their MGP. In Lewisham and Deptford especially the midwives highlighted the satisfaction and support gained from working in a group of midwives who shared a similar approach to providing midwifery care. In all MGPs when things got tough at work the majority of midwives cited their colleagues in the MGP as a main source of advice and support. Highlighting the importance of support from colleagues, an Ashford midwife told us: 'There is no difference to the way I practise except support from my colleagues which I never had before. Someone to help me clear up! It didn't matter if I'd been up all night and all day, nobody cared.' It also underlay the reasoning of the Deptford midwife who felt that the MGP was '...less disruptive to my life. I know the women I'm working with. Knowing the midwives and being on the same wavelength is a rarity and absolutely lifesaving.'

In Lewisham and Ashford midwives commonly felt that they had achieved greater autonomy and more flexible working and also took more responsibility for the women. As one Lewisham midwife put it: 'More flexible working and not feeling persecuted for it. Freedom of being able to plan your day how you want and the amount of time you are able to spend with the people ante and postnatally.'

Most midwives in all three groups felt that their role as a midwife had been enhanced by working in the group practice. They felt they were using their midwifery training more fully and that working in the MGP had extended their skills and experiences. A frequent comment was that this way of working enabled them to provide more holistic care. Comparing the MGP with her previous experience of community midwifery, one explained: 'There is a tendency for midwifery to be compartmentalised. Community midwifery is largely postnatal. In the group we provide total overall care to everybody and it can make a difference during labour and birth for the women.' Another emphasised: 'My role as a midwife was ill-defined before – all to do with hospital procedures and fragmented care. I never saw how women gained or not from what I did. Before it was all to do with large throughput.' It was common for midwives to feel that this greater involvement had increased their confidence and made them more assertive in their dealings with other professionals including GPs and obstetricians.

Identifying the most rewarding aspect of working in an MGP, the majority of midwives cited the ability to give total care to women, along with getting to know the women and their families and ensuring that women had a positive experience of pregnancy. Their comments frequently echoed the Lewisham midwife who said that for her the most rewarding aspect was, '...to be able to give the care from the beginning to the end and to hear the women say "I'm glad we did it this way".' In Deptford, midwives also highlighted their satisfaction with being able to achieve their mission of offering the type of service that some of them had previously provided as independent midwives to a wider range of women, and within the NHS. In this MGP establishing the women's health resource was seen by the worker responsible for this activity as 'fundamental and crucial to *Changing Childbirth*'.

Challenges

Working in the MGPs had also presented midwives with a range of demands and challenges, some of which were difficult to sustain. For some the entire experience of working this way had been taxing: 'The whole thing has been a challenge. Trying to tie it in with everyday life. To keep home and work separate is a challenge. It is a 24-hour involvement.' A number of specific challenges were also identified and these frequently mirrored concerns that midwives had expressed at the outset.

Impact on family life

To a considerable extent reservations about longer hours, tiredness and the amount of time on call had been borne out in practice and had impacted on family and social life. Most of the midwives in Lewisham and Ashford and half in Deptford had found the work rota and on-call arrangements demanding. They talked about the difficulties of juggling home and professional life and the demands that were placed on relationships.

One Lewisham midwife felt particularly strongly: 'It's demanding. It disrupts family life. I miss seeing my husband and children. It's difficult to plan family gatherings. They accepted it at the start but can we sustain it? The family needs continuity too.' Another commented: 'My poor husband and son have had to suffer. I must say if you have a demanding husband you're heading for a divorce. The job is very demanding. The family has to support you. It's not everybody's cup of tea. It's not fair on people with young children.' Where young children were involved, midwives frequently referred to the cost of arranging childcare to cover the unpredictable hours away from home.

In Ashford some of the midwives felt that a change in the duty rota part way through the monitoring period had eased the demands of on-call and its impact on family life: 'It's better now. At the start it was 24 hours on-call. Now we have split the day into two parts. All within the team now have family commitments other than husbands. We can't say we are single and idealistic.'

It became apparent, and was borne out by midwifery managers, that in some instances midwives were opting to place additional demands on their time over and above the duty rota. This was reflected in the remark heard in Lewisham: 'I don't find the on-call demanding. It's when you are not on-call and people expect you to come out that it is difficult. If someone rings you at 2 am it is difficult to say no. We divert our phones at night. However, when we are not on-call we have said you can ring the lead midwife and give her the option for delivery.' Explaining this, one midwife referred to a sense of 'guilt' experienced if they did not go out to 'their own women'.

Responsibility

Whilst offering women greater choice and taking more responsibility for their care had lead to greater job satisfaction, it had also been awesome in some respects. In Lewisham we were told: 'You become not just their midwife but their companion, almost a psychologist. All the barriers come down. Women build up this trust – it's daunting.' In Deptford there was reference to: '...being drawn on to your last ounce of energy. Having to make decisions when you are the most responsible person.'

Group dynamics

The start of study interviews indicated that group dynamics would be an important factor in determining both midwives' satisfaction with their job and the achievements of the MGPs. Midwives' initial comments revealed that working in a group practice held the potential for providing a stimulating, supportive network, but there was concern that it could also create tensions and conflicts. So it proved. While working within a group of midwives was often cited as a source of satisfaction and support, group dynamics were also singled out by six of the midwives (2 in Lewisham and 4 in Deptford) as perhaps the most challenging aspect of the work.

In Lewisham tensions within the group were linked to the way in which the group had been assembled, with some midwives being recruited to the scheme and midwives not necessarily choosing to work together. Initially in Deptford there were some tensions and a group counsellor was consulted. The problem was resolved part way through the monitoring period when the composition of the MGP changed. One of the midwives who remained with the group explained: 'We had problems last year because people had different ideas about how the practice should work. People from different backgrounds. Inter-personal difficulties are now resolved. We have a stronger base we are all happier with. Last year one or two midwives were not happy about the direction and the stress of an insecure future.'

In all MGPs some midwives felt they were working harder than others on the business side and this could be a source of tension. Whereas they were likely to feel that colleagues were slow in volunteering for certain administrative or promotional activities, their colleagues were just as likely to feel that they were not given the opportunities to get involved or be heard.

Any tensions within the groups should not, however, be exaggerated. Virtually all of the midwives felt that generally they had worked well as a group. Minor differences in style (for example, the extent of contact with women, preferences on where to see women) were recognised but were not perceived to be in conflict with the overall shared philosophy of the group. Differences in skills and experience were viewed positively, with midwives welcoming the opportunity to learn from each other. At its most basic, an Ashford midwife concluded: 'It's had its ups and downs but essentially works well. We're all different and do things a little differently. If we communicate, problems do not arise.' More positively a Deptford midwife referred to '...a lot of give and take and we're very good at listening and supporting each other and because of our shared approach it's easy to discuss things.'

In looking at group dynamics it is important to note that none of the MGPs had formally nominated a group leader. However, it was observed by a senior midwifery manager for one of the groups that, '...there is by default... there comes a natural leader out of any group'. This was also an issue in the early days for Deptford, with one of the midwives remarking that, while there was no group leader and the midwives were self-employed on an equal professional basis, '...however, some people have more power in making decisions, whether this is because of a louder voice or experience.'

The majority of midwives preferred to use the term 'coordinator(s)', and it was apparent that in each group this role was performed by one or more of the midwives, as explained by a Lewisham midwife: 'There are coordinators but that's not really team leaders. Coordinators make sure the group practice is running smoothly, but they're not in control. It was a group decision to appoint them.'

Regular group meetings, usually on at least a weekly basis, were an essential forum not just for discussing aims, exchanging information and reviewing caseloads and practice, but also for defusing group tensions. In Lewisham one midwife referred to the importance of these meetings for 'getting rid of frustrations', although a colleague was more dismissive of their function which she reduced to '...a time to shout at each other. If you don't go you don't see other midwives unless you bump into each other. The time for argument. I find them boring and don't find them useful.'

Working with other professionals

At the start of the study some midwives had concerns about how they were perceived by hospital midwives and how their working relationship with GPs and consultant obstetricians would evolve. In practice midwives both within and between MGPs seemed to have had quite varied personal experiences.

General practitioners

Particularly in Lewisham and Ashford, midwives were likely to talk about their experience of building up confidence and trust with local GPs. It helped if they had already worked in the GP's surgery: 'They are supportive because they know me. I've been there four years. One GP said if we had a new midwife who wanted to practise this way he would be more reserved. They are confident in my competence.' Where trust had been established with GPs, midwives felt that GPs were approachable and supportive. This provided the opportunity for exchanging information and views on professional practice and sharing knowledge about the woman and her family.

It was common, however, for midwives in all three practices and particularly in Deptford to point to weaknesses in their working relationship with local GPs. There was talk of hierarchical relationships, poor communication and lack of interest or even hostility on the part of GPs to the MGPs. Midwives thought the most likely reasons for these attitudes were that GPs feared losing contact with women during pregnancy and that for them this represented a break in continuity of their overall care for women as their GP. As a Lewisham midwife explained: 'GPs are feeling bereft. Losing control. They like contact with pregnant women. It is a happy event. They want to see positive outcomes.' Several midwives said that their women did not necessarily want to see the GPs during their pregnancy: 'Mums want more than a quick fumble, dipstick in the urine and a blood test.' Some GPs were also thought to be wary about home deliveries, not interested in obstetrics or worried about losing their skills.

In Deptford a specific observation was: 'The fact that we are radical, independent of the authorities, self-employed has terrified them.' Some of the more extreme reactions were recorded in this MGP and in the early days of the study we were told: 'We have had... no negative feedback from anyone except GPs. They're being quite aggressive, shouting down the phone saying, "What right have you got to talk to my women?" I think they feel threatened.'

Consultant obstetricians

A similarly varied picture emerged in relation to consultant obstetricians. In each of the MGPs it seems that the midwives had established a good working relationship with at least one consultant obstetrician but had found it difficult to establish a rapport with others. Where a good relationship had been established midwives tended to feel that the consultant obstetrician was more accessible than before, as illustrated by this Lewisham midwife: 'I would never have rung up a consultant obstetrician before because the hierarchy was so pronounced. They now value our midwifery role.'

Reinforcing this point a colleague in this MGP confirmed: 'If we have someone with a problem we can ring them up or take the woman to them. It's good in terms of their views. They see us more as a team looking after the women.' Also in this MGP the observation was made that '...the women love to see a working relationship between professionals rather than conflict.' Similar comments were voiced in Ashford and Deptford, with one of the Deptford midwives explaining why a good relationship with consultant obstetricians was easier to establish than with GPs: 'It's very clear cut. We know our boundaries. We know when to refer women. No blurred edges like with GPs.'

There tended to be an over-dependence in each of the MGPs on a small number of supportive consultant obstetricians. In relation to other obstetricians midwives alluded to poor communication and insufficient contact stemming largely from a lack of interest in the MGPs on the part of the obstetricians. They were seen to be set in their ways and wary of midwives extending their territory. In Deptford the comment was made: 'They don't know us very well. There is a tendency to make assumptions about home births and attitudes. They think we're whacky midwives doing things that aren't completely safe. It's because they don't know how we work.'

Hospital midwives

Few strengths were perceived by the MGP midwives in their working relationships with hospital midwives, although in Deptford in particular the

MGP midwives emphasised that they tried to make hospital midwives feel valued and to work with them. In each of the three MGPs it was reported that hospital midwives had tended to view the MGP midwives as an elitist group who did not wear uniforms and whose role was not fully understood. As one Lewisham midwife commented: 'We are seen as a sacred group. Hospital midwives are more rigid.'

There was concern that in some cases hospital midwives had either refused to care for MGP women, or on the other hand had treated them without informing the MGP midwife. In Lewisham it was remarked: 'To begin with there was confusion around communication. Hospital midwives have not called the project midwife and they delivered... We now liaise with the ward staff by using a link worker.' Lack of understanding about the role and objectives of the MGPs had also contributed to jealousy from other midwives which had been experienced in Lewisham and Ashford: 'I think a lot of midwives in here still don't know what JACANES means. We get lots of snide remarks.'

The lack of willingness to help on the part of hospital midwives was particularly apparent on the postnatal wards and one of the Deptford midwives pointed out: 'If women are in hospital they are in there for a reason – like risk. I would need a camp bed to give "ongoing vigilance". Hospitals are staffed to give vigilant care to women with problems.'

While some of this reserve or hostility was put down to a lack of understanding and confusion over respective roles, the MGP midwives also highlighted the possibility that hospital midwives felt threatened by change. Illustrating this point we were told: 'They feel we are JACANES – so get on with it. There is an attitude problem on both sides. People don't like change. Some hospital midwives feel threatened by the concept of *Changing Childbirth*. It's not what they want to do but if we succeed they will have to change too.' Similarly it was observed in Lewisham that: 'Initially they put up barriers. Perhaps they were saying "We're not going to work like this, give up our free time, drop social and domestic commitments".' It was recognised by midwifery managers that if *Changing Childbirth* was to be implemented successfully there would need to be better integration between hospital and MGP midwives, and to achieve this they would have to work as hard with those midwives who remained within the hospital as with the MGP midwives.

Assessment of success

At the end of the monitoring period around three-quarters of the midwives considered that their MGP had been very successful and, with one exception, the rest felt that they had been fairly successful in achieving their aims. They based their assessment on a range of criteria. All the midwives identified user satisfaction as the main criterion, particularly whether the women would come back to use the service again. As one midwife summed up: 'That's the whole point of a woman-centred service.' Specific comments in this area included 'empowering women' and ensuring that they had 'positive birth experiences'.

The midwives' own motivation and job satisfaction was also identified as an important factor, along with low sickness rates. It was crucial, one Lewisham midwife felt, '...that the midwives want to continue working in this way and don't leave.' Empowering midwives was a specific comment made by one of the midwives, but a warning not to stray beyond professional boundaries was sounded by another: 'We have our 10 pointers, the things we should have achieved... and that the whole thing hasn't moved away from the Midwives' Rules and Code of Professional Conduct – whether you're still working within your parameters.'

Clinical and labour outcomes were also seen as indicators of success: 'Physical outcomes – can it be demonstrated that clinical outcomes are as good?' Other important indicators included breastfeeding rates, and the perceptions of other professionals.

Asked what was the most significant achievement of their MGP, midwives in Lewisham tended to refer to the continuity of care provided. A factor highlighted across all groups was 'survival'. As an Ashford midwife emphasised: 'Getting through it. For the group to have stayed together after all the stress we've been through. No-one has left or given up.' In Deptford the biggest achievement cited by some of the midwives was getting funded at all as a direct provider unit within the NHS.

Problems experienced

All but two of the midwives felt that their MGP had experienced some problem or difficulty which had made it less successful than it might have been. In reflecting on these difficulties they cited things that they felt should have been done differently in establishing and running the MGPs.

Shared concerns centred around pressure of work and tiredness and in some instances it was felt that this had affected the quality of care that the MGP was able to give. An excessive caseload was identified as a problem in JACANES before JACANES II was set up and the process of setting up this second MGP was also singled out as a factor 'interrupting the flow of success'. The size of the caseload was also a problem for Lewisham midwives and we were told that there needed to be a mechanism for limiting the caseload for individual midwives.

Group dynamics which we have already discussed was a central weakness for some midwives, particularly those who left the Deptford practice. As we have noted, in Lewisham this issue was related to recruitment issues. Midwives reiterated points made earlier that they did not choose whom they wanted to work with. In this MGP some of the midwives felt that team selection criteria and the grading policy should have been different. The latter point was also raised by Ashford midwives. A point made was that in practice there was not enough difference between the F and G grade midwives to justify the difference in pay.

Problems with defining roles and communication with other professionals, particularly with hospital midwives, has already been discussed. Lack of management support from some quarters was mentioned by some of the midwives in Lewisham and Ashford as a weakness which had impacted on the way the MGP had developed.

Another observation related to the amount of work involved in setting up the midwifery group practices, and it was emphasised in both Ashford and Lewisham that SETRHA had asked for protocols at very short notice.

Lack of administrative systems and support was also identified by some of the Lewisham midwives. As one complained: 'The paperwork we have to do is extra on top of giving the women the care. Since we are so mobile and we have not got a permanent office as yet we have to keep a filing system in our heads and it is very difficult.' This was exacerbated by the time and effort demanded of midwives to fill in the forms for the evaluation.

In Deptford the perceived weaknesses were largely associated with insecurity of funding and inexperience of the contracting process. One of the midwives described the issue as: 'Funding and the problems arising from that. Meeting the right people. Getting hold of them, talking to them on their terms. Trying to understand the process and how money is provided and how long it takes.' They were concerned about creating a demand among women, and expectations on the part of GPs through networking, and then not being able to book women because they had no funding. This had evoked strong feelings as one of the midwives illustrated: 'We are immensely frustrated and I personally feel quite betrayed. I feel that the Region led us a merry dance really.' A general feeling in this MGP was that fighting for funding had detracted from providing the service and had created a hiatus in bookings.

In commenting on what they felt should have been done differently, the main argument in Deptford was that there should have been more assistance with setting up the funding. One of the midwives spoke for all in the group when she said: 'I want to talk about the money. It's absolutely vital. Pilot projects should be supported properly. If it's intended to run for two years it shouldn't be funded for less.'

Replication

In terms of testing out and evaluating a model of care the majority of midwives thought that it was important that the pilot MGPs had been set up in three different geographical areas and were perhaps catering for different needs. Commenting on replicability one of the midwives said: 'Wherever you set up it's got to be tailored to geographical and community needs... All the three projects are different. We're all approaching things from a different angle. None of us have the complete answer but you can combine lessons from the three.'

Two-thirds of the midwives thought that the model of care that they were piloting could be transferred to other areas, but several added strong caveats that the caseload would need to be smaller and on call time would need to be reduced. Pay and grading issues would also need to be reviewed along with job share arrangements. As one midwife observed: 'Unless these changes are made the expectations are unrealistic and cannot be sustained.' The midwives who said the MGP was not replicable in its current form similarly gave as reasons the fact that the caseload was too large and that on-call time was excessive. Essentially the majority of midwives were in fact agreeing that the *framework* of the MGP was transferable, but not without amendments to reduce caseloads and to contain on-call time. The Deptford midwives also made the point that any future MGP set up on similar lines to theirs would need greater security of funding than they had experienced.

There was genuine concern in all MGPs, however, that midwives would not universally want to work in this way. As an Ashford midwife commented there was a risk that the model was 'not acceptable to a wide enough selection of midwives' and that good midwives, particularly those with young children, might be lost because they could not fit in the style of work with home circumstances and family commitments. The issue of motivation and training was also raised by one of the midwifery managers as a potential obstacle to expanding the MGP model across the service as a whole. Her concern was that many of the midwives already practising in hospitals and the community would not be as enthusiastic and prepared to work the long and unpredictable hours required to meet the expectations of the MGPs as the midwives who had opted to become involved in the pilot projects.

Unintentionally this point was also captured by one of the midwives who said that the MGP was proving very successful: 'Because it's what the clients want and it's what we want to give the clients, and because it's a pilot scheme you're going to work harder to make it successful. We're hoping to make it so successful that all the other midwives in the area will want to do the same thing.'

Chapter 8

General practitioners and consultant obstetricians

Interviews took place with 38 general practitioners (GPs) in the three pilot sites. In Lewisham and Ashford, all these interviews were with GPs in the practices in which midwives from the midwifery group practices (MGPs) were based. We refer to these as 'host practices'. For the Deptford MGP, we contacted GPs from all the GP practices who were given as the source of referral for women on the forms completed by the midwives. For the sake of simplicity, we have referred to the three sets of GPs as the Lewisham, Ashford and Deptford GPs, although they were not necessarily based so closely within these geographical areas, particularly in Ashford and Deptford.

We interviewed all 11 GPs (5 men and 6 women) from the three host practices in Lewisham. We interviewed 15 GPs (12 men and 3 women) of the 19 GPs in the five host practices in Ashford. In Deptford, we achieved interviews with 12 of the 18 GPs we approached (5 men and 7 women). The responses from the GPs in Deptford clearly differed from those of the host practice GPs, most markedly because they had no experience of having members of a midwifery group practice based in their surgeries. Indeed, most had had little contact with the Deptford MGP midwives and two said they had had no contact at all. However, their views and experience are of interest, partly to compare with those of GPs who were working closely with MGP midwives and partly to highlight the reaction of a variety of GPs whose patients were using the Deptford MGP.

The average age of the GPs was 43, with little difference between the three areas. GPs under the age of 45 accounted for nearly three-quarters of those interviewed in Lewisham, in Deptford for over two-thirds and in Ashford for nearly two-thirds.

The average length of time they had been working as principals in general practice was 11 years, with those interviewed in Ashford having been principals rather longer on average than in the other two areas. All but two of those interviewed were working as full-time principals.

Maternity care provided by GPs

Rather surprisingly, not all the GPs interviewed were included on their Family Health Services Authority's (FHSA) obstetric list. All the Ashford GPs were, but 3 of the 11 Lewisham GPs were not (one man and two women). All but one woman of the 12 Deptford GPs were on an FHSA obstetric list.

We asked the GPs about the range of maternity care they personally provided to women attending their practices. All but one of the GPs (a male Lewisham GP) said they provided *antenatal care,* and all but one (a male Lewisham GP) provided *postnatal care.* The picture for *intrapartum care* was very different, however, with only a quarter (3) of the 11 Lewisham GPs (2 men and 1 woman) providing such care, compared with just over half (8) of the Ashford GPs (7 men and 1 woman) and a quarter (3) of the Deptford GPs (1 man and 2 women).

None of the GPs in any of the areas provided intrapartum care in a *GP maternity unit.* 3 of the 8 Ashford GPs and 1 of the 3 Deptford GPs who provided intrapartum care did so in a *combined consultant and GP hospital unit,* which none of the Lewisham GPs did. All 3 of the Lewisham GPs, all 3 of the Deptford GPs and all but one woman among the 8 Ashford GPs who provided intrapartum care said they provided this care at home.

Five of the 38 GPs had personally delivered a baby in the previous 12 months – three had delivered one baby (all home births), one had delivered two babies (one normal delivery at home and one instrumental delivery in a hospital unit) and one had delivered three babies (one normal delivery at home and two normal deliveries in a hospital unit).

In the previous twelve months, three of the GPs had personally performed one perineal repair and two GPs had personally performed two perineal repairs. The average length of time since the GPs in general had had training or retraining in perineal repairs was nearly 13 years, and the average length of time since they had had training or retraining in delivery was 12 years. The range of time since training or retraining was wide, and was clearly related to the age of the doctor.

Choice of lead professional

One of the crucial issues we were asked to examine was the extent to which women were offered choice – most particularly choice of care, of carer and of place of birth. The question of whether, how and by whom women are offered choice of 'lead professional' is of fundamental importance to many of those involved in implementing *Changing Childbirth.* But, as we have seen, different players have different interpretations, not only of the concept of choice but also of the concept of 'lead professional'.

So we asked the GPs whether they themselves personally offered all women who came to them for advice about their pregnancy and maternity care the choice of having a midwife, GP or obstetrician as their lead professional. The answers were by no means straightforward. Nearly half of the Lewisham GPs (5), over half of the Ashford GPs (8), and two-thirds of the Deptford GPs (8) said that they did personally offer choice. Of these, 1 Lewisham GP and 3 GPs from both Ashford and Deptford said that this would include women with a high risk pregnancy.

Most of the GPs in Lewisham and Ashford who did not personally offer all women a choice of lead professional said that this was because the midwife offered women the choice. One Ashford GP and 4 Deptford GPs said that they encouraged all women to have both midwife and GP input.

There were clearly tensions arising with some GPs who said that it was the midwife who offered the choice. A Lewisham GP who was concerned about the extent to which GPs were being excluded from antenatal care explained: 'I have left that discussion since the project began. I've just said that the midwife will be seeing you later on. We didn't seek to exercise power – there's an awful lot of power with someone offering care. I didn't offer choice – with the understanding that the midwife would be offering those choices. They can't have been doing it.'

Another Lewisham GP stressed the need for close contact with the midwives, although his comments underlined the need for trust and continuing exchange of information between GPs and midwives: 'Even with high risk they would be offered a midwife, but we would expect the midwife to say, "No way Jose – I'm not having this."' He was not completely certain that the midwives were following his recommendation.

The main reason given by GPs who did not include women with a high risk pregnancy among those to whom they offered a choice of lead professional was their view that the obstetrician should be the lead professional in such cases.

Some GPs were prepared to take a pragmatic approach with women who 'insisted' on midwife or GP care when they would prefer them to have hospital care, but others stated their unhappiness, like a woman Deptford GP: 'I'm very concerned about people feeling that nature is best and patients making demands which put them at risk and involving the health professionals in situations where they might feel otherwise professionally.'

An Ashford GP spoke of the need for careful negotiation with some patients: 'If they are happy with us and then I say they need a specialist, they trust me. If I bully them they won't trust me.'

There was clearly increasing ambivalence on the part of some host practice GPs who had entered the project on the understanding that offering a choice of lead professional was a good thing, but had found that they were not able to interpret how this choice had been offered. Much, of course, related to the concept of 'lead professional' which, as we have seen, was open to so much interpretation.

Lead professionals

We asked the GPs what they considered to be the value of having a 'lead professional' in relation to maternity care. There were some variations among the areas. Two-thirds of the Lewisham GPs and nearly the same proportion of the Deptford GPs thought that the main value was that women knew to whom to turn first, compared with one third of the Ashford GPs.

Over half the Deptford GPs, one third of the Lewisham GPs and a quarter of the Ashford GPs thought that the main value of a lead professional lay in having continuity or consistency of care.

A quarter of the Ashford GPs, one fifth of the Lewisham GPs but only one of the Deptford GPs thought that having a lead professional meant that clear clinical responsibility could be attributed. Others thought that it was useful in coordinating and disseminating information.

Some thought it had value for several reasons, like a Lewisham GP: 'One has to consider the advantages, particularly if it is a well-known figure to the woman. It should lead to a better transfer of information, for example in terms of safety because one person feels they are responsible. If you look at perinatal deaths, failures in communication are a very common problem. It's also important for the women to know whom to contact when they are concerned or worried.'

However, some GPs in each area thought it was not a practical concept for a variety of reasons, mainly because the complexities of maternity care required a team effort or because one professional was not available all the time. And some GPs were concerned throughout the interview about the question of accountability: 'Legally there can only be one person who can be responsible and I'm it! I'm still responsible.'

Even where GPs acknowledged the value of having a lead professional, many put forward caveats, some of which were practical – 'It's practical on weekdays. It's unpractical out of hours of weekends, or if the person is on holiday when the delivery date comes...' – while others were more complicated, as this Lewisham GP pointed out – 'I have had problems because I'm not quite sure of the line of responsibility when there is a problem with the pregnancy. Do I ring the midwife or the obstetrician? I do feel that the midwife should be informed. There is a kind of blurring if there is an obstetric emergency or problem.'

A Deptford woman GP was more doubtful about how the concept was put into practice, particularly in the case of midwifery-led care: 'It's a good theory, but it doesn't address the long-term issue of health throughout a lifetime. Although in theory, one person is responsible, when it comes to the moment of crisis, often the midwife isn't available. Often patients ring us for advice, and, because there isn't enough communication between the midwife and us, we haven't a clue what we're dealing with.'

There were concerns in all areas among GPs that the concept of 'lead professional' could lead to a deterioration of overall care for women, and that there was a danger of dogma interfering both with professional standards and with common sense. A Lewisham GP thought: 'It's to do with a power struggle between professionals. The government is siding with the midwives. As long as there is good quality care it doesn't matter. Women with severe mental or physical problems get poorer care because it is no longer shared with the doctors.' His views were echoed in Ashford: 'No way can one person be responsible. Childbirth cannot be a separate entity. It's a complex matter, both medically and socially and everybody should be involved, including the midwife.'

As we found among the midwives, there was a lack of clarity among GPs about what 'lead professional' meant, and there is no doubt that some clarification would be helpful. At the moment, there is a danger that it could lead to unnecessary competition among professionals about who is 'in charge' of maternity care at a time when the ethos of *Changing Childbirth* is that women should be given greater choice and independence.

Midwife-led care

We have seen that the midwives themselves were not in agreement about the definition of 'midwife-led care', and these differences were reflected in the views of GPs. There were differences between the three areas in their interpretation of what it meant. One third of the Lewisham GPs, over half the Ashford GPs and four-fifths of the Deptford GPs thought that it meant that midwives were the lead professionals, giving virtually all the care, leaving the GPs to do the first booking and postnatal check. Most of the rest of the GPs thought that it meant that midwives were responsible for most of the care but should refer to the GP or consultant obstetrician if there were complications.

Three GPs from host practices thought that midwifery-led care meant care which excluded GPs, while others thought that it could work, provided the care was consistent with that given by GPs and that it was recognised that GPs were ultimately accountable and responsible for their patients.

There was clear evidence of increasing tensions between some of the host practices and the way midwifery-led care had evolved in Lewisham and Ashford. A Lewisham GP summarised his views: 'My experience of it is that we don't see the women in pregnancy. The way it's been interpreted is that GPs do the booking – the main channel of entry into the system. We write a letter to the Focus midwives – and then we see a set of notes when they need a postnatal visit. We all suggested that that doesn't give us much involvement.'

These worries were echoed in Ashford: 'As it's practised by JACANES, it means the midwife does everything until there's a problem. They don't let us in until there is a problem. And sometimes these girls have never seen a doctor. It's midwife only care.'

In Deptford, there were strong reservations about a system in which contact with the MGP was even more removed from the GPs. One woman GP said: 'We're responsible for *all* our patients *all* the time, and we don't like not knowing what's going on.' Another Deptford GP was particularly concerned about how midwife-led care could lead to the exclusion of all other professionals and could lead to a confusion of roles and inappropriate advice: 'The midwife is the contact point for the women in question, but they shouldn't act in complete isolation from other health professionals. I would like to have a significant role. I don't want to see a pregnancy test and then do a baby check after a home delivery and know there has been an awful lot in between. If we have midwife-led care we have to have accessible midwives, who communicate with ourselves and are non-confrontational. There has been poor communication and conflicting advice particularly about neonatal immunisation which has been controversial. It can be very unsettling for the women to have conflicting advice.'

The warning signals flagged up here were reinforced when the GPs were asked in what circumstances they thought that midwife-led care was appropriate. Around one third of the Lewisham and Deptford GPs, but nearly two-thirds of the Ashford GPs, thought it was appropriate if there were no high risk factors, while around a quarter of the Lewisham and Deptford GPs but few of the Ashford GPs thought it appropriate if the woman wanted midwifery-led care and there were no contra-indications. Around one fifth of the GPs in all areas though it appropriate in all cases provided the GP was not excluded. Only one GP – in Ashford – thought it ought to be available in all cases for anyone who wanted it, while one GP – also in Ashford – thought it was not appropriate in any circumstances. He commented: 'Under no circumstances. I was the one who supported this idea. But what is happening now is I don't see the patient at all – unless she's dying!'

The main message from the GPs was that midwifery-led care was appropriate as long as due recognition was given to the physical and mental condition of women, that midwives recognised the boundaries of their expertise, and, most important, that the GP was not excluded in midwifery-led care. There was clear evidence from these interviews that the way in which the MGPs had functioned in practice had led to a situation in which many of the GPs had felt not only that their relationship with their patients had been adversely affected but also that their own input had been marginalised, in many cases to the detriment of the overall care received by the woman during her pregnancy, leaving aside the question of whether the GPs might be deskilled or less satisfied by having a much-diminished contribution.

It appeared that some of the problems identified by the GPs could have been alleviated by better systems of communication and sharing of information between the midwives and the doctors, as an Ashford GP highlighted: 'I'm not against the midwife being the lead professional. It's the exclusion of the GP that's the problem. We've been effectively excluded in this scheme. I'm not getting a look-in at all. We're not getting the information. We're asked to write the letter to the hospital, but we're not asked to see the patient. There is no ongoing exchange of information.'

In one host practice the GPs had insisted from the beginning that they saw the women at least twice during their pregnancy: 'My partners like to keep in touch with their patients. They like to see them twice so that their relationship keeps going. They are going to be caring for the mother and baby long term. I don't think the patients should feel that they have been abandoned just because they are pregnant. I have access to their medical history.'

But time and again in these interviews, there was a clear indication that GPs were sad to lose contact with women during an important period of their lives, as expressed by a Deptford GP: 'I do share the worry expressed by other GPs that the GPs could be pushed out. I don't personally want that because I enjoy providing obstetric care and I think it would be a shame if it stopped.' Her concern was reflected in another form by another Deptford GP: 'I don't think there should ever be an instance where your GP doesn't know you're pregnant. I don't think there's a scenario where no medical input is a good thing. Equally, no midwifery input would be a bad thing.'

Direct access to midwifery care

We were interested in the views of the GPs on whether they thought that women should be able to go direct to a midwife to arrange maternity care without seeing a doctor first. The GPs interviewed were by no means adamant that they should be the first port of call for pregnant women, and over half of the GPs in all areas thought that women ought to be able to have direct access to midwives. However, many of these added certain provisos, particularly concerning agreed protocols and the continuing exchange of information between GPs and midwives.

A Lewisham GP who thought a woman ought to be able to go direct to a midwife was quite clear about the circumstances in which this should happen: 'Only if we sit down and work out the protocols first. If she goes straight to a midwife, what about other problems such as epilepsy or schizophrenia or drug addiction. How can the midwife advise? So it is appropriate for some and not for others.'

An Ashford GP thought it appropriate if there was trust between a GP and midwife: 'She's an individual who's specialised in midwifery care, which is more than you can say for the majority of GPs...' But another in the same practice was less sure: 'This question has been superseded by events, it's too late to pose such a question. The stable door is closed.'

A Deptford GP summarised the views of a number of GPs: 'I don't see why not, but it would be the only situation where an aspect of women's medical care doesn't involve a GP. A main aspect of the GP system is that they know the history of a woman. It is a shame if a woman goes off for nine months and the GP picks up the pieces afterwards. Therefore I think the woman should have direct access if they want it but I am sad about it. I am a "family" doctor.'

These views were reinforced by the GPs who thought that women should not be able to go direct to a midwife to arrange maternity care. The main reasons they put forward were that GPs needed to know what was happening to their patients, that the midwife needed the GP's cover and knowledge of the woman's medical history and because they felt, very strongly in some cases, that pregnancy and birth were part of family medicine and the 'cradle to the grave' care that they felt that GPs should give.

A Lewisham GP expressed the views of many about the importance of 'family' medicine, but also highlighted the need to put pregnancy into the whole spectrum of care: 'We expect to care throughout their lives and enjoy the involvement. I feel strongly that GPs should be involved in antenatal care. But it is a small part of their lives. There is a risk of nine to twelve months of special care – for example home visits and mollycoddling. It is not possible to provide this level of care for anyone else. Our practice takes pride in antenatal care. The immunisation level is high – they trust us. Without this involvement of the GP in antenatal care, ongoing family care is more difficult.'

An Ashford GP agreed: 'We are looking after them 24 hours a day, 365 days a year. Why shouldn't we be part of maternity care? It's not fair on us.'

Some of the Deptford GPs had the greatest reservations, as a woman GP pointed out: 'We are the first they phone when something goes wrong. We have to know what is going on. We have to be involved in some way. It has to be a working partnership.' Another Deptford GP was doubtful: 'It is difficult to say. If they were registered with me and I didn't know they were pregnant and something goes wrong, who's responsible?'

Another Deptford woman GP felt unhappy about the idea of direct access to midwifery care by women: 'Midwives don't have the full medical records – and if they did have them, they don't have the training to understand them.'

It was the perceived lack of overall medical expertise and training among midwives that concerned a number of GPs in all areas, as an Ashford GP pointed out: 'We should know every aspect of the patient, not just the obstetric/gynaecological past, but heart problems, lung problems, housing problems, brain problems, husband problems, children, parents – and two years in midwifery clinics doesn't cover that. Why do we go for years to medical school?'

Choice of place of birth

Over 90 per cent of the Lewisham GPs thought that all women should have a choice over the place of birth, compared with two-thirds of the Ashford and Deptford GPs. However, most of those who thought women should have a choice qualified this with the proviso that there should be no risk to the mother or baby or that the woman should be fully informed of all the possible options and of all the implications of home births.

It was interesting, however, that most of those who thought women should have a choice over place of birth interpreted the question as one which was aimed at establishing whether women should have a choice of having a home birth. A Lewisham GP noted: 'Every woman should have a choice, but it's our duty to advise women of the safest place to have a baby. Most women are reasonable and understand. For many women a home birth is a fulfilling experience which they shouldn't be denied, but disasters do happen.'

Some women GPs in all areas had definite views both on the availability of choice but also on their own preferences, like this Ashford GP: 'They have a perfect right to have a baby at home. It's wrong to over-medicalise a normal pregnancy. *I'd* never contemplate having a baby at home, because of the risk of foetal distress, and facilities are very limited at home.' A Deptford woman GP agreed: 'I wouldn't like a home birth myself. For high risk women they need to be fully informed about the advantages and disadvantages. They have to be aware of what is and is not available – for example the flying squad – and weigh up the information. If they still want it then I have no objections to that... It depends on the situation and resources though. We had one woman who lived on a river boat.'

The extent to which women should have the sole choice of place of birth concerned a number of GPs, like this Lewisham woman GP: 'I think she should have a choice, but so should the doctor. It puts the doctor in a difficult position. If something goes wrong they are going to feel so responsible. A woman's choice should be tempered by the doctor's choice.'

Over a quarter of the GPs thought that not all women should have a choice over the place of birth, mostly because of the risk of obstetric complications. Only three doctors said they were against home births in principle, often combining this with fears of litigation or concerns about the adequacy of back-up services. An Ashford GP said: 'I don't like home births. I don't want to be involved in them – mainly for legal reasons. I don't want to be involved in the case-law that decides it.' A Deptford GP agreed: 'Home deliveries is a no-no. In the old days perinatal and maternal mortality were high in the case of home births. We would be going backwards. I believe in natural things, but there are limits to everything.'

Another Ashford GP said: 'I am extremely unhappy about home confinements. A patient can die within minutes from a postnatal haemorrhage. You see the bed fill with blood – it does still happen. We aren't equipped for home confinement. We don't have an adequate ambulance service. We don't have the obstetric flying squad any more. It's a disaster waiting to happen.'

We have seen from the interviews with midwives that some of the Ashford GPs were said to be against home births, but while the GPs themselves usually cited risks and safety factors, the midwives had implied that some GPs lacked the obstetric skills themselves. There was clearly a breakdown in communication between some of the GPs and the MGPs on the subject of home births in all areas, and again we emphasise how essential it is for discussion and agreement on protocols and practice before midwifery-led practices are embarked upon.

There were also concerns among GPs, whether they agreed that all women should have a choice of birth or not, that it was not always possible to inform a woman fully of all the potential risks in a home delivery. The question of what constitutes 'informed choice' is clearly an issue to which those implementing *Changing Childbirth* must return time and again. In all the interviews we conducted with professionals and women we touched on different aspects of it, but the answer remained elusive and we return to it in our discussion of findings.

Women holding case notes

We found that all the Lewisham and Ashford GPs reported that all women receiving maternity care in their practices held their own case notes throughout their pregnancies, while this was reported by two-thirds of the Deptford GPs.

Most of the GPs were in favour of women holding their own notes, mainly because they felt it involved women in their own care and led to better relationship with professionals, because it meant that the notes were in one place and available for different professionals or in an emergency, because it offered a single record which was a good coordinating mechanism, and because they were less likely to get lost than in a hospital, for example. As a Lewisham GP observed: 'The patients are more reliable than the hospitals in producing records.'

With such overwhelming support for women holding their own notes, it was surprising to find any dissenting voices, but one GP found the A4 folder inconvenient while another thought that women might lose their notes. Two of the Deptford GPs noted that it was not the practice in their local hospital for women to hold their own notes.

How GPs became involved as 'host practices' to the midwifery group practices

We were particularly interested in the experiences and views of the GPs in Lewisham and Ashford within the practices which had agreed to act as 'host practices' to the midwifery group practices. We asked a series of questions to elicit their views on a variety of subjects, to see what lessons could be drawn for others who were thinking of setting up similar models of care and organisation, while recognising that there were differences within the areas themselves, not only between GP practices but also among the individual midwives. There were also, of course, differences within GP practices.

We found a striking difference between the areas in how the GPs thought they had originally become involved as host practices. In Lewisham, more than half of the GPs interviewed thought they had become involved because they were sympathetic to midwifery-led care, while this reason was volunteered by only one of the 15 Ashford GPs. As many as one third of the Lewisham GPs and two of the Ashford GPs did not know how they had become involved.

On the other hand, over half the Ashford GPs said that they entered by default or that it was presented to them as a 'fait accompli' – a situation reported by none of the Lewisham GPs. One GP in Lewisham and a quarter of the Ashford GPs had become involved through their own existing midwives being part of the proposed MGP. It is, of course, possible that this was interpreted by some Ashford GPs as a 'fait accompli'. The question of interpretation was important, but it had certainly led to some ill-feeling among Ashford GPs. One commented: 'Our midwife retired and we got landed with the midwifery group practice.' Another was equally critical of the process: 'We lost our highly-valued and trusted midwife and the new ones were involved with JACANES. So we entered by default.' And others spoke of a lack of choice: 'The scheme was decided upon and introduced without consultation with the doctors.'

There were clearly potential problems from the start in introducing midwifery group practices in such a way, and it is probable that some of the uneasy relationships we observed in the Ashford area between GPs and midwives could have been avoided with better planning and introduction of the MGP schemes.

We asked the GPs what had interested them most about becoming involved as a host practice. Over half the Ashford GPs said that they were interested in *Changing Childbirth* and improving the patterns of maternity services. Nearly half the Lewisham GPs said they were most interested in the guarantee of continuity of care, while others in both areas were interested in seeing how the concept of midwifery-led care would work in practice and increasing the involvement of women in their own care. Around one fifth of the GPs in both areas said that nothing interested them particularly about the schemes, either because they were not consulted before it started or because they were not much involved in antenatal care: 'I wasn't interested because I wasn't consulted – it was imposed.'

Some GPs in both areas noted that they had been initially attracted by the scheme but had changed their minds since: 'We thought it was a good idea at first – midwifery-led care. Now we see the patients less and less.'

It was not perhaps surprising that the GPs had had some reservations about becoming host practices, although this was much more marked in Ashford, where three-quarters of them (11) had had reservations, compared with under half (5) of the Lewisham GPs.

The main reservations expressed by the GPs were that they would lose continuity of care with their patients, and that they would not be able to establish bonding or a good relationship with a woman in the antenatal period which they considered to be important for the postnatal period and subsequently. In Ashford, nearly half of those expressing reservations had been worried about losing skills or seeing their skills transferred to other professionals, while a quarter had concerns about standards of care in an untried system. Only two doctors (one in each area) mentioned a potential loss of income.

Some of the women GPs had had the greatest reservations. A Lewisham woman GP said: 'I had huge reservations. One was about losing control and knowledge of the women and a very valuable part of general practice. I also had concerns about the medico-legal side of who is responsible if people don't turn up and something goes wrong.' Her concerns were echoed in Ashford by another woman GP: 'I was concerned that it might decrease our involvement – and it has done. We were very involved with deliveries. It has diminished our relationship with our patients, and as a result they lose out as well.'

Professional responsibilities

In looking to the future, it is clearly important to establish protocols on who should be responsible for what aspects of care in a variety of circumstances. We asked the GPs how the respective responsibilities of GP, group practice midwife and consultant obstetrician had been agreed upon in their practices, with particular attention to protocols.

Again there was a marked difference between the areas and within the areas. In Lewisham, half the GPs said that there had been individual agreements between the MGP and the GPs, while the rest of the GPs said that they had no knowledge of any protocol or had no knowledge of how the respective roles of GP, midwife and consultant obstetrician had been agreed upon. In Ashford, one third of the GPs said that the agreement had been imposed upon them, and that neither they nor the obstetricians had been consulted, a quarter said they had no knowledge of any protocol, two thought there were no clear-cut directives on responsibilities, while one thought it had emerged through individual agreements between the MGPs and the GPs. On the other hand, three GPs said that there was a protocol set out and available.

Although much depended on how the GPs interpreted what was meant by protocol or agreement, it was clear that there was a degree of muddle in how the respective roles of GP, midwife and consultant obstetrician had been agreed upon, and indeed there was considerable doubt about whether they had been agreed upon in most of the practices. This must be a cause for concern. A woman Lewisham GP spoke of evolution in determining roles and responsibilities, underlining the need for proper planning and negotiation before schemes begin: 'Nothing was written. I don't remember any discussion about it. We did discuss the GPs' role at home births. We renegotiated with the midwives so that we could see the clients twice during the pregnancy because we weren't seeing them at all.'

In Ashford, the resigned acceptance of a 'fait accompli' pervaded many interviews, as one GP noted: 'We had protocols – but we had no say in it. I don't know who drew them up.' Another GP was more critical: 'There were pages and pages of documents, but they weren't consultative. Comments were invited at a meeting at JACANES, but the general impression was that it didn't matter what we said. A lot of work had gone into it already – and it was too late to change.'

Changes in maternity care provided by GPs since MGPs set up

Many observers will be looking at the models of practice demonstrated by the three midwifery group practices, and none more keenly than GPs. What changes to their own practice had the GPs within the host practices experienced over the 15 months or so in which the MGPs had been running at the time we interviewed them, and what did they feel about them?

We asked first whether the range or extent of maternity care personally provided to women by the GPs had changed since the midwifery group practices had been set up. Over 80 per cent of the Lewisham GPs and over 90 per cent of the Ashford GPs reported changes, with only two Lewisham GPs and one Ashford GP noting no change.

The main change reported in both areas was less input by GPs into antenatal care, but one Lewisham GP and four Ashford GPs reported that they now had *no* input into antenatal care and that the pilot had resulted in an exclusively midwife-led care scheme. Three of the Lewisham GPs and two of the Ashford GPs said that the main change had been that they now did far less or no intrapartum care. On the other hand, two GPs reported more input in following up home deliveries and one GP did more postnatal visits than before.

The descriptions given by the GPs of their changing practice showed serious disquiet, as a Lewisham GP noted – 'It's changed out of all proportion. I don't see pregnant women any more. I don't attend home births any more. We can't cope with the on-call commitment and the midwives are keen to cope on their own.' There was little doubt that many of the GPs were surprised and concerned at how quickly things had changed, like this Ashford GP: 'I don't seem to be having a role in it. I don't see the ladies alternately with the midwife as we used to. My skills are deteriorating and I'm only two years out of hospital.' His concerns were reflected by another: 'There's far less GP input since JACANES. You don't lay your hands on pregnant abdomens which could have long-term snags and loss of skills. You quickly lose skills in medicine if you don't use them.'

In one Lewisham practice, the GPs had quantified the dramatic changes: 'In the event in the first six months we had 27 per cent of the antenatal consultations we had before. There would be two or three of us doing it and we might have seen five or six each – the midwives ten. In the first six months we were seeing one or two each. The midwives hardly had a clinic. There were many clinics where the midwife just popped in to say "Hello" because she was doing most of the visits at home.'

How did the GPs who had noticed a change in their roles feel about it? Nearly three-quarters of them in both Lewisham and Ashford said that they were unhappy at their lack of involvement and lack of opportunity to build up relationships with women. One GP in Lewisham but nearly half the Ashford GPs said they were unhappy about their loss of skills. Two GPs were concerned about practical problems that had occurred with the midwives, while three expressed concerns about safety or being called in only in a crisis. Only one doctor (in Ashford) expressed unqualified satisfaction with the changes, while two GPs in each area said that they were mostly happy, but were concerned that they might be being by-passed. Three doctors said that the patients liked it.

The comments made by the GPs are of considerable importance in assessing how best to implement *Changing Childbirth,* since the involvement and support of GPs can undoubtedly affect the extent to which these models of care are replicable.

A Lewisham woman GP summarised the views of a number of her colleagues: 'I miss seeing the pregnant women, but I accept that seeing them at home is less "medical" for them. I have mixed feelings about missing home births. It's a commitment, but I do miss it. It's a good bonding experience.'

There was certainly a view that the antenatal period offered a chance for both women and GPs to establish a good relationship which formed a basis for future care in a more relaxed atmosphere than was often possible when dealing with sick patients, as a woman Lewisham GP explained: 'I miss the antenatal care. It kept you very much in touch throughout the pregnancy. You get to know them very well when you see them when they're fit and not coming to see you only when they're ill.'

The lack of involvement in antenatal care also had implications for intrapartum care, as an Ashford GP explained: 'Having previously had a lot of involvement in intrapartum care, now I'm expected to do home deliveries for mothers for whom this is my only involvement. I'm aware that decisions are being made inappropriately by midwives for midwife care, which should be made by me. I feel we're providing worse care than before, and I personally am becoming deskilled to the point where I won't feel comfortable in giving the whole range of maternity care in future. And I think that's very sad.'

Sadness and frustration were words which were used frequently in these interviews with GPs to describe their feelings about the changes they had experienced which they thought had led to their relationships with patients suffering. A woman GP was in no doubt about how she felt: 'I hate it. I see some postnatals and sometimes I'm faced with a lady with whom I've had very little relationship. I feel I'm losing my skills and losing the opportunity to keep abreast of what's coming along now.'

And a male Ashford GP was even more concerned about the far-reaching implications of what he saw happening: 'The concept of family medicine, the cradle to the grave concept – the bonding between GP and family – that's in jeopardy.'

Assessment of success of the midwifery group practices

We were interested to see what criteria of success the GPs would use in judging the success or otherwise of the midwifery group practices. As we found among the midwives themselves, the overwhelming majority of GPs said that user satisfaction was the most important criterion. However, two-thirds of the GPs said that clinical outcomes or clinical audit would be among their criteria, which was less frequently mentioned by the mid-wives. The midwives themselves were more likely to mention the morale of the MGP as a whole as a measure of success, while this was regarded as a criterion by less than half the Lewisham GPs and one third of the Ashford GPs. Similarly, the midwives often mentioned their own motiva-tion and job satisfaction as a criterion, while none of the GPs singled this out as important in measuring the success of the MGPs. On the other hand, over one fifth of the GPs thought that GPs' job satisfaction was an important criterion, while none of the midwives even mentioned this. And two of the Ashford GPs thought that the relationship between GPs and the MGPs was an important criterion – another factor not mentioned by mid-wives.

The GPs were much more likely than midwives to mention specific clin-ical outcomes as criteria that they would use in judging the success or otherwise of the MGPs, including infant and maternal mortality and mor-bidity, safety issues, numbers of Caesareans, number of episiotomies, maternal mental health, immunisation rates, breastfeeding rates and rates of home and hospital births. The question of cost-effectiveness was men-tioned by two GPs in each area.

Given the high level of critical comments made by the GPs in both areas, it was perhaps surprising to find that nearly half the Lewisham GPs

(5) rated the midwifery group practices very successful according to their criteria and over one third (4) thought it had been successful. One fifth (2) felt unable to comment. The Ashford GPs were more reserved, with only a quarter (4) rating the scheme successful or very successful, nearly half (7) rating it fairly successful, 2 saying that it was not really successful and 2 saying that they did not know.

Why did the GPs think the scheme had been successful according to their criteria? Four-fifths of the Lewisham GPs said that the patients seemed happy, a view shared by less than half the Ashford GPs. Other reasons for success in both areas mentioned by a handful of GPs were thought to be the continuity of care offered by the MGPs, the accessibility of the midwives and the professional competence of the midwives. A quarter of the Ashford GPs were rather more grudging and attributed a certain level of success to the fact that there had been no serious clinical failures.

On the negative side, one third of the Ashford GPs and one fifth of the Lewisham GPs said that the lack of communication from the midwives had made the scheme less successful than it could have been, while others thought that it had resulted in less involvement of GPs, problems in defining roles and responsibilities and exhaustion of midwives. One GP thought it had been a waste of money and resources.

The questions we asked related to the criteria that GPs would apply to judging the success of the MGPs, and a Lewisham GP indicated the complexity of applying a variety of criteria to assessing how successful the pilot had been: 'The women have loved it. I think it has been extremely successful from that point of view. They have got to know the midwife and she has been there at delivery. I think a percentage have the antenatal care in their own homes. There is a greater continuity of care. I don't think we – the GPs – are as enthusiastic because of our decreased contact with the women. I think relations with the midwives are not as good as they used to be. It's becoming "them and us" and they look extremely knackered most of the time.'

An Ashford GP was rather more circumspect: 'Some patients like it; some clearly don't. We get calls from patients who haven't been able to get through to the midwife - patients we haven't seen.' And it was this lack of contact with patients which dominated the interviews with many of the GPs in host practices, however much they might have thought the scheme successful in other ways: 'Those of us who've had training are probably unhappy to have no role. Probably very anxious too, because of a grey area on who's ultimately responsible for the patient. If there's a consultant referral, I have to refer, and frequently I've never seen the patient.'

What should have been done differently?

Three-quarters of the Lewisham GPs (8) and nearly 90 per cent of the Ashford GPs (13) thought that, looking back on the history of the midwifery group practice, things should have been done differently.

The main factors identified by the GPs were that there should have been more GP input and consultation at the outset, that there should have been better communication during the project between GPs and midwives, and that the overload on midwives should have been foreseen. In addition, two Lewisham GPs thought there should have been clearer directives on responsibility and one thought there should have been a preliminary survey of patients' wishes.

But who should have taken responsibility for doing things differently? In Ashford, GPs tended to think that the midwives' managers should have taken on the task, while in Lewisham, GPs were more likely to think that GPs themselves should have been more proactive. In Ashford, responsibility was also laid with the working party who defined the protocols and 'everybody involved', while in Lewisham two GPs thought that the regional health authority should have played a stronger role.

A Lewisham GP saw the pilot project as part of a wider debate which could lead to unnecessary inter-professional rivalry: 'I see it as a political power struggle. I see it as a push by the midwives to take over. I would have sat down with the midwives and decided which patients are appropriate for midwife care and which are appropriate for shared care. But it saves the government money this way. It's a much cheaper option. It's doing the midwives in. They just can't cope with it. Also the pregnant women don't get the companionship of others. It's a shame. They lose their support group.'

In Ashford, there was considerable discontent about the extent to which the GPs had been 'excluded' at the beginning and had not been consulted since. A woman GP said: 'There should have been more GP input in the beginning and more asking GPs how involved they'd like to be – by the midwifery group practice.' Another woman GP agreed: 'We should have been given more choice, and communication lines should have been more firmly established at the start. There should be stricter guidelines about the paperwork – informing the GPs of births and how results are to be dealt with and so on.'

Another Ashford GP said that communications were 'atrocious': 'We need to meet; we need to discuss. It would be nice to still have involvement, say three or four meetings with the patient and midwife during pregnancy. There should be more shared care really.'

In analysing these accounts it was sometimes difficult to understand not only how the lack of communication between GPs and midwives could have arisen but also how it had continued for so long. One of the practices had taken matters into their own hands and had insisted on some changes, but it had taken time for this to happen, and relationships with the midwives remained rather strained. In other cases, relationships and trust appeared to have deteriorated over the course of the pilot project, and it seemed that a lot of goodwill on the part of the GPs had evaporated, possibly beyond repair. Careful assessment should be made of how this had happened and what steps should be taken if similar schemes are to be implemented to ensure that host GP practices do not feel themselves to be ignored, marginalised and deskilled simply because of lack of planning and communication.

Knowledge and experience of midwifery group practices

We wanted to establish to what extent the host practice GPs knew of the other midwifery group practices taking part in the pilot project. We were also interested in learning not only whether the GP practices whose patients were using the Deptford midwives knew anything about the other MGPs but also their views of the Deptford MGP.

Among the 11 Lewisham GPs, we found that just over a quarter (3) had heard of the JACANES MGP in Ashford and that two-thirds (7) had heard of the SE London (Deptford) MGP. Among the 15 Ashford GPs, we found that two-fifths (6) had heard of the Lewisham Maternity Focus Group and that the same number (6) had heard of the SE London (Deptford) MGP. Among the 12 Deptford GPs, we found that two-thirds (8) had heard of the Lewisham Maternity Focus Group, just under one fifth (2) had heard of the JACANES MGP in Ashford, and, surprisingly, only 10 of the 12 said that they had heard of the SE London (Deptford) MGP, despite prompting by the interviewer. They were, after all, selected because their patients were being given care by the Deptford MGP.

We asked the Deptford non-host practice GPs what they considered to be the main aims of the MGPs they had heard of, whether they provided any information about them and whether they had referred any women to them.

Those who had heard of the Lewisham MGP thought that its aims were to provide continuity of care and midwife-led care and there were single mentions that they aimed to offer a choice of home birth and a known midwife at delivery. None of them gave any information to their patients about the Lewisham MGP and none had referred any women to it. The Deptford GPs who had heard of the JACANES MGP knew nothing about its aims and, not surprisingly had not referred patients or given any information to patients about it. Of the 10 Deptford GPs who said that they had heard of the Deptford MGP, 3 said they understood its main aims were to offer continuity of care and midwife-led care, 4 thought it was to focus on disadvantaged groups, such as homeless people, poor clinic attenders, drug addicts and those with HIV, 3 thought it was to focus on ethnic minority groups, particularly Vietnamese, 2 thought it was to provide an alternative model of midwifery care, while there were single mentions for providing care for high-risk women, to offer a team approach and to encourage breastfeeding.

6 of the 10 GPs said that they offered information to women about the Deptford midwives. This ranged from information only to those who wanted a home birth or 'alternative medicine' (3), the provision of leaflets (2), description of the type of independent group with NHS funding (2), and single mentions for verbal information on address and telephone number, and information to those who might fit the criteria of needing extra support.

A male GP said: 'I describe the form of the service, their aims and intentions, and ask if the woman would like to know more. The women who go there are generally self-selecting and it does seem to go on a class and educational basis. Perhaps they *should* be targeting people from the groups who, unfortunately, are the most reluctant to use it.'

And a woman GP described what she did: 'I've handed their leaflets out – to someone I thought would fit their criteria – a girl who didn't fit into conventional medicine and wanted to have a home birth. I thought they would be what she is looking for.'

Only 7 of the 12 Deptford GPs said that they had ever referred any woman to the Deptford MGP – 1 male GP and 6 women GPs. Considering that all 12 were interviewed because they were listed as being the GPs of women using the Deptford MGP, this was surprising and could be a cause for some concern, in that some of the other 5 seemed unaware that their patients had used or were using the Deptford MGP.

One GP said she made perhaps one referral a month, but all the others said they referred less frequently and qualified their remarks by saying it was mostly or only at the patient's request or only in special cases where a home birth was requested or where extra care was deemed necessary. One GP said: 'We have referred some women quite late – at 36 weeks or more – first time mums who were frightened or needed extra confidence.'

Another GP who said he had referred added by way of explanation: 'Three have self-referred. I have seen them during pregnancy usually when they asked for a certificate to see if they are fit to fly. This emphasises the problems of communication. One other – I gave her a leaflet and she contacted them herself. A lot of our intelligent middle-class women live in the Greenwich area and the care offered there is extremely good.'

Impact of midwifery group practices on existing maternity service provision

We asked the GPs the same question we had asked the midwives about whether they thought that the services offered by the midwifery group practices had improved maternity services for women locally. Although the midwives had almost unanimously agreed that they had, the GPs were by no means so sure.

Two-thirds (7) of the Lewisham GPs, three-fifths (9) of the Ashford GPs and one third (4) of the Deptford GPs thought that their respective MGPs had improved maternity services for women in their district. Women GPs were marginally more likely than men GPs to think that the MGPs had achieved improvements.

The main factor cited by the Lewisham GPs as an improvement was the increased continuity of care and personal attention which the Lewisham MGP had brought. There were single mentions of the convenience of home visits for the women, a known midwife at delivery, a named midwife, that patients liked it, less wasted time in hospital visits, more opportunities for a home birth and better help and support in breastfeeding.

In Ashford similarly, the increased continuity of care was thought to be the most important improvement, with rather more acknowledgement of having a named midwife. Again, there were single mentions of increased choice for women and less wasted time in hospital. In Ashford there were also comments about the greater appropriateness of midwives for routine antenatal care, thus freeing the consultants for high risk patients, and praise for highly motivated midwives, a high standard of care and the possibility of longer antenatal consultations.

The Deptford GPs were more limited in their response, but three GPs thought that the Deptford MGP had offered access to high quality care by an alternative route, and there were single mentions for continuity of care, more time, higher standards of midwifery, parentcraft and antenatal classes and 'private' care on the NHS. A woman GP commented: 'It's widened the choice for women who would want that type of care but couldn't afford it before. I'm not sure they are reaching the deprived groups specified in their contract or the ones they would like to reach. They are not doing it because there is a lack of information in the community about them.'

But, as we have seen, a substantial proportion of GPs thought that the MGPs had not improved maternity services to women locally. The main reason for this view in both Lewisham and Ashford was that the service was no different from before and that it had always been a good service. In Ashford we heard more comments on the dangers of an increasingly fragmented service and the view that the MGP service was too restricted to midwife only care.

The main reason given by the Deptford GPs for judging that the Deptford MGP had not improved maternity services in the district was its failure, in their view, to reach its target groups of disadvantaged women and that it was used mainly by self-selecting higher income group women. There were other concerns, including a perceived encouragement by the MGP for women with unsuitable home circumstances to have home births, the discouragement of infant immunisation and a feeling that the MGP was too 'political' and 'anti-doctor'.

A woman GP identified a number of problems that she had observed: 'The way they like to practise – very pro-home delivery, a very nice patient-friendly service, but the very patients they target are the very worst candidates for home delivery. Also, it's unfair because it isn't being used for women in need, but by people who'd heard about it and fancied getting a good service on the NHS. If you want to have special funds, those people they target are the very ones who need to be encouraged to have a hospital delivery. There's a political problem here, an anti-doctor feeling, 'empowering the people' sort of thing. But the advice of these midwives wasn't just restricted to the maternity area, and we found almost all the mothers who'd been on their books actually refused vaccinations for their children. Why should the NHS fund a service which undermines itself? If people want the kind of service they offer, they should pay for it.'

Her views were echoed by another woman GP: 'I am seriously worried about their impact on what the women believe. Those midwives are strongly against immunisation.'

Strengths and weaknesses of midwifery group practices

We explored further with the GPs what they saw as the strengths and weaknesses of the midwifery group practices compared with other existing arrangements for midwifery care. Throughout this study we were looking for ways in which the model of care provided by the MGPs were seen to be providing lessons for others.

Main strengths

Among the Lewisham GPs, the main strength of the MGP was thought to be the continuity of care provided by the midwives, together with their dedication and commitment. It was also thought by a quarter of the GPs to be liked by patients. Other factors, each mentioned by two GPs, included the professional skills of the midwives, the accessibility of the service, the time given by the midwives, and the saving in hospital time, and single mentions of the adaptability of the midwives and the convenience of home visits for the patients.

The community base of the MGP was stressed by two GPs. One said: 'It's inappropriate for healthy women to be traipsing to the hospital when they don't require this. Hopefully this would free up obstetric schedules to deal with problem pregnancies.' Another thought that the MGP's strengths were: 'The trust and relationship between client and midwife, the convenience of home visits and avoiding cluttering up the hospital clinics. It's very time-consuming to see the obstetric registrar, and unnecessary for a lot of the time.'

Similarly in Ashford the main strengths of the MGP were thought to centre on the continuity of care, dedication and commitment of the midwives concerned. Again their professional skills were mentioned by one third of the GPs, while there were mentions for the accessibility of the service, patient satisfaction, the advantages of midwives working in pairs, the enhancement of primary care, and cost effectiveness.

The majority of the Deptford GPs thought that the motivation and commitment of the Deptford MGP was its main strength, while 5 of the 12 said that patients liked it, 3 mentioned the time given by the midwives to women, 2 spoke of the advantages of working in pairs and there were single mentions of women feeling 'special', the offer of an alternative model of care, accessibility to deprived groups and the 'autonomy' of the MGP.

A woman GP in Deptford summarised what she saw as the strengths of the Deptford MGP: 'It focused on "feelings" quite a bit. It makes every woman feel special. I haven't yet met anyone who has regretted using them. They give them time. They listen to them. They are reliable. They give continuity of care.'

Another woman GP reinforced this view somewhat wistfully: 'They give continuity of care, the personal touch – and time. They've got far more time than we have and that's only possible because of the inequity of funding. It would be nice if we all had that sort of funding. Dream on!'

Main weaknesses

The main weakness in the MGPs as a model identified by the Lewisham GPs was the danger that they marginalised GPs and worked in too isolated a way. Three-quarters of the Lewisham GPs mentioned this and it was clearly of great importance to them, as had been evident throughout most of the interviews. In addition, over one third of the GPs said that the midwives had too heavy a workload. Other comments include fears about fragmentation of family medicine, midwives making decisions outside their knowledge base, midwives making too many unnecessary home visits and the cost of the service being too great.

A Lewisham GP summed up the views of many of her colleagues: 'It's work intensive for the midwives and they get very tired. We have insisted on seeing the patient and I would be very unhappy if we hadn't done so. We want a shared midwife/GP role.'

The problem of marginalisation of GPs was again the main weakness identified by most of the Ashford GPs. One third of them thought the midwives were suffering from overload – 'It's stretched the lead midwives a lot. It's taken its toll...' – and a similar proportion thought there was danger of diminution of family medicine and bonding with patients. Other weaknesses related to potential deskilling of GPs, exclusion of GPs from the enjoyment of maternity care, the lack of accountability of the midwives and the management of the midwives.

A woman Ashford GP had given a lot of thought to the problems: '1) There's a lack of accountability. It's a group of six midwives and I don't have a clue who, for example, is going to look at a dodgy blood test or whatever. 2) There's a danger of GPs losing their skills, and at the end of the day we're responsible for the whole list for the total care of our patients. 3) There's a weakness in GPs not having a say in which midwives are allocated to patients. 4) There's fragmentation – difficulties with note-keeping and computer records for us. The midwives don't use our computer, so there are incomplete records. 5) There are difficulties in getting hold of the midwives.'

In Deptford, the weaknesses of the model were thought to be more varied, mainly because few of the GPs had had much contact with the MGP, so that the impact of potential marginalisation of GPs caused by midwives taking over their role was less clearly apparent than among host practice GPs. However a quarter of the GPs noted that there was a weakness in that GPs were not kept informed about what was happening to their patients. Other weaknesses mentioned by at least two GPs each were thought to be inappropriate selection for home births, inappropriate advice about childhood immunisation, the 'wrong' people (i.e. middle class) benefiting from the MGP, too many unnecessary home visits, adverse effects on family medicine, and single mentions of poor relationships with other professionals, too much emphasis on home births, the isolation of the MGP and too heavy a workload.

There were some sharp criticisms by Deptford GPs of the Deptford midwives. A woman GP observed: 'Firstly, they are too self-involved. They are a bit isolated. They have set up good links with hospital units for emergency services and hospital births, But they have a philosophy which means that they are not very objective in the way in which they handle situations which could affect their judgement – for example risky factors around birth and post partum... We've had problems in the postnatal period. There is not sufficient liaison with GPs about babies who are not thriving. We have had problems with liaison with us on when does "normal" become "requiring medical attention". There is an inability to involve other professionals, not having had experience of working with GPs. GPs don't want to be involved with them.'

Another woman GP noted: 'We have had anxieties about their commitment to childhood immunisations, whether they adhere to national guidelines on Vitamin K for babies and the extent of choice given to women to have their perineum sutured after tears. It is all left very much to maternal choice and this is sometimes not informed.'

Another woman GP spoke of her fears: 'It's inequitable – the wrong people are benefiting. It's too political – issues of a strong home birth movement which can put heads in sand over the risks involved. And it's the worst time for home births – I'd be happier if there was a really good flying squad and a fully named midwifery team – for example re postnatal haemorrhage and the need to put them on a drip quickly. We've spent 24 hours a day learning to do that and midwives haven't.'

Replicability

To what extent did the GPs feel that the model of the midwifery group practice in their area could be transferred to other districts in its present form? Two-thirds of both the Lewisham and Ashford GPs thought that the model was transferable, but most added a number of provisos. Half the Deptford GPs thought that the model offered by the Deptford MGP was transferable, but again most added qualifications to their answer.

The main reason that GPs thought that the model of care offered by their local MGP was transferable was that the patients liked it. However, the provisos added were similar to those put forward by the GPs who did not think that the model was replicable elsewhere. The main qualifications cited by both groups were that:

- there should be better communication between midwives and GPs;
- there should be appropriate and effective management of the MGPs in place;
- the respective roles and responsibilities of GPs, midwives and consultant obstetricians should be laid down in protocols and agreed in advance;
- there should be checks on whether protocols were being followed;
- there should be less stress and overload on the midwives;
- it needed highly dedicated and committed midwives who might not be universally available;
- it should be properly funded;
- it should be adapted to local needs;
- it might not be possible to ensure a known midwife at delivery;
- it might not be possible to replicate evening home visits;
- it was recognised that it was an expensive model of care;
- it could lead to fragmentation of care if GPs were not in favour of it;
- it might only be suitable for deprived areas with special needs;
- duplication of effort should be avoided;
- it could produce a two-tier service.

Among the GPs who thought that the model could be transferred to other areas, a Lewisham GP expressed the views of a number of his colleagues: 'It is excellent where GPs are not prepared to provide antenatal care. I just think I'd personally prefer more input. I think there's a need for a more flexible approach to antenatal care and a recognition of the long-term perspective the GP has. It should be a primary care/community based *team* rather than midwife-led. There should be an equality of roles.'

Another Lewisham GP thought that it was particularly suitable for deprived areas: 'The more underprivileged the area, the more valuable it will be. When people are in a tough environment, they miss their clinics, but the midwives can go round to their house. If people have got four kids and no transport, it's difficult to get to a clinic. I think underprivileged areas are key areas and it's very valuable.'

A Deptford GP thought that one of the problems with the Deptford MGP was that it had not attracted people in underprivileged groups: 'It attracts upper middle class articulates. Their mission statement says that 75 per cent should come from various target groups, but I get the impression that they are providing free care for upper middle class women who could afford private care.'

But a Deptford GP who thought the model of midwifery group practices was transferable in principle urged a realistic approach: 'Here you have the pick of independent midwives and the cream of Lewisham midwives in the Focus Group going over the top. It is not replicable within the normal resources available and it gives false ideas. It is dependent on the energy and personalities of the midwives involved.'

Another Deptford GP who thought the model was not replicable spoke of the problems she thought would be involved in attempting to transfer the Lewisham MGP model: 'I went to one of their presentations. They had a ridiculously high number of women – I think they said 98 per cent – delivered by a named midwife. That is not replicable. They had midwives working on their time off. It's not civilised and there are not enough hours to do this. They do lots of home visits in the evening. That is again unrealistic and unsustainable. They're providing a Rolls Royce service for some women. It's not right and we should look at the service for all women. Women are prepared to go to the clinic rather than getting midwives to always see them at home. One of the midwives said her job satisfaction had gone right up and one of the GPs said his job satisfaction had gone right down.'

And it was the continuing worry of creating a two-tier system, of fragmentation of the maternity service, of marginalising or excluding GPs from maternity care, of overloading midwives that exercised the minds of many GPs at the end of this interview when asked if they had any additional comments about the midwifery group practice pilot projects.

There was no doubt that the midwives in the MGPs were mainly seen as highly dedicated, committed and hard-working. But some GPs were concerned that this was by no means a universal phenomenon and that caution should be exercised in assuming that midwife-led care could be implemented in general. A Lewisham GP noted: 'What it has done is to select a group of very dedicated midwives. It has done nothing to improve the interpersonal skills of midwives in hospitals. I would like to see it lead to improved standards of midwifery.'

But among GPs in all three districts, there were fears of women 'falling through the net', of decreased contact by GPs with both women and midwives, of lack of clarity on roles and responsibilities, and potentially of less good care for women, particularly if good liaison and working relationships between midwives and GPs was not established.

There were strong reservations expressed by the Deptford GPs in particular, as a woman GP noted – 'I would feel it's nice to be consulted rather than just getting a letter to say, "I'm taking over this case".' Some of the GPs were particularly concerned about whether women were always well enough informed to make some of the choices they were taking: 'My worries are over the selection of patients. I question whether some of these women and their partners really do know enough about what is involved to question the opinion of specialists. And when it goes wrong, it goes disastrously wrong. I'm happy enough if we can agree a selection of patients and if we can agree where individual responsibility lies.'

A woman Deptford GP agreed: 'I'm very concerned about patients making half-informed decisions. The repercussions can be immense. People are getting the impression that doctors are making problems and that there aren't any risks and everyone is going to end up with a healthy baby. I have an anxiety that some midwives have very militant and political views.'

And another Deptford GP summarised the views of many GPs in stressing the need for a holistic approach: 'It's important to distinguish between continuity of care in pregnancy and longer term care. This treats pregnancy as a one-off item and not as part of the life cycle. Pregnancy and childbirth are part of a whole life experience of a couple. It should not be removed from general practice care... Pregnancy is a very important time for health promotion – particularly diet and alcohol – and time to consider the socio-economic problems of a child coming into the family. Where GP services are failing there is a place for midwife-led practice, but I see this as an admission of failure. I would like to see any money available spent on improving primary care and not on the fragmentation of the service. Bring the midwives and specialists into the team. Let's have integrated care.'

And it was this desire for an integrated service, with team working, shared goals and defined responsibilities that was a constant theme in the interviews with GPs in all three areas. An Ashford GP spoke of the need to look at maternity services within the framework of a primary care led health service: 'Highly specialised professionals devoted to maternity services should give strength, but I'm not sure if they should do it alone. I'd rather that it stayed integrated in the family doctor team. Now, instead of integrated maternity services, we've got a separate group. It's going against all the trends in primary care.'

Consultant obstetricians

Consultation with a consultant obstetrician by women booked to deliver in hospital

To what extent did women booked to deliver in Lewisham Hospital and the William Harvey Hospital see a consultant at least once in their pregnancy? None of the consultants reported that this was a routine procedure, mainly because it was not considered necessary or feasible. In one hospital, it had been the practice of two of the consultants, but pressure of numbers had resulted in the discontinuation of this practice: 'It's impossible now with the number of deliveries – I do over a thousand a year. The intention is there but it's practically not possible. But I go through the notes and write to the GP on *all* patients.'

In some cases, consultants said that women were frequently booked under the care of a midwife and even if they were booked with a consultant they might not see him if they were low risk. In other cases, consultants said that they would see a woman if she requested it or if the GP or midwife thought it necessary.

Views on existing service provision

All the consultants thought that the present maternity services, excluding the midwifery group practice projects, met the needs of women in the district, but most added some qualification to their comments.

One consultant thought that most needs of most women were met, but was concerned about whether the quality of services was as uniformly high as he would have liked: 'The present services meet the majority of needs. Most have a choice about place and type of birth. A concern is the increasing number choosing to have elective caesareans. We are seeing a patient-led increase in planned epidural caesareans. People asking for a high-tech solution.'

This comment seemed a far cry from the view held by so many of the midwives that women were requesting 'natural' births and home births.

For two of the consultants, the biggest problem at present was ensuring continuity of care. One said: 'If you mean in terms of providing a safe and patient-friendly service, then overall we do meet the needs of the women. If you mean are we able to give women everything they may want or need, then no. But then, no-one does. For instance, for the vast majority of women the biggest deficiency is the inability to provide continuity of care at the midwife level.'

One of his colleagues agreed: 'We have gone a long way to improve care, but it would be better if women could see the same doctors or midwife throughout. At present, women see the same group of doctors and midwives, but not the same person necessarily.'

Lead professional

The concept of 'lead professional' in relation to maternity care was as unclear to some of the consultants as it had been to the midwives and GPs. One consultant, however, had no doubts: 'I'm of the opinion that the consultant should be the lead professional in all cases – as team captain who decides the policy.' Another consultant thought that it was the person with ultimate clinical responsibility: 'This person has traditionally been the consultant, who had carried the ultimate responsibility, to whom a woman can come with a problem that other carers haven't been able to help with – the lead clinician able to provide continuity of care.'

Others were not so sure, and were divided on the value of having a 'lead professional' in relation to maternity care. One consultant said: 'I don't like that term. It's got to be a team effort. One individual cannot take total responsibility. But in most circumstances it would be a midwife. It's better to use the term "link professional". That person may not be the person who makes the decisions and is accountable.'

Another said that it was important that women had someone to whom they could relate and whom they could trust: 'The lead professional needs the skills to allow the patient to communicate. In theory it's more likely to happen if the person has a continuous focus of reference. But some women find it easier to talk about intimate things to someone who is not familiar.'

Midwife-led care

There was some lack of consensus over what midwife-led care meant. Some consultants were concerned that it might be interpreted as midwife only care, which was a matter of concern to them. All consultants thought that in all cases midwives should refer appropriately. One commented: 'It's where the midwife is the lead, the "principal", professional from the outset to the conclusion, and only refers for extra advice and assistance where she deems it necessary. She uses her full panoply of skills.'

When did the consultants think that midwife-led care was appropriate? One had definite views: 'I think the midwife is the person who should be looking after normal uncomplicated pregnancies. The midwife is the ideal person to do that. But that doesn't mean that she should be on her own. She has links to GPs and consultant obstetricians, but she is not leading as such. She liaises with the appropriate people and makes judgements, so is autonomous in her own right, in normal cases; but she must recognise what is normal and abnormal. It's appropriate in totally uncomplicated, low risk pregnancies.'

One of his colleagues in another hospital agreed: 'It's more appropriate for low risk, as was the intention of the original protocol.' But a consultant in the same hospital thought the discussion had become politicised: 'The argument is that women now are more healthy. Another argument is that it works in Amsterdam, so transfer it here. I would prefer a woman to register with her GP, for the GP to pass her to the community midwife for booking and initial investigation. Then for her to come to the hospital once and be reviewed by the medical team. Then for the hospital to see her again twice more. I'd like the hospital practice and the GP to say she's normal and the midwife will supervise her. Now the only time we see them is when they are on the ward in labour.'

Direct access to a midwife

The consultants were split on the question of whether a woman should be able to go direct to a midwife to arrange maternity care without seeing a doctor first. One said: 'She's entitled to. It's a free country. If a patient wishes to approach a midwife only, as she can do legally and the midwife is obliged to take her on, then the midwife has responsibility until that patient is referred to a GP or a consultant obstetrician.'

But three of the consultants were against it, particularly since they felt the GP should be involved. One consultant echoed the reservations felt by so many of the GPs interviewed: 'There may be odd occasions when it is appropriate, for example, if there's a bad relationship with the GP. But in general terms, by-passing the GP is not a good model... It sends the wrong message to the GP: that the woman undervalues him. It damages the GP/patient relationship. She will need to see him later as the family doctor. She would also miss out on being referred by the person who knows more about her medical history and health. He can give her the initial screening and ask her what model of care she wants. Don't short-circuit the GP.'

A consultant at another hospital was equally concerned: 'It's always worrying that women want to go to a midwife to the exclusion of the GP. There may be circumstances in relation to health that the women doesn't want to mention to the midwife, putting her in a difficult position, and therefore creating problems further down the line. It's worrying that there could be significant breakdown in the relationship between the GP and the woman.'

Choice of place of birth

The consultants were again split on whether women should have a choice over the place of birth. Although three of them thought that women should have a choice, they all felt that the choice should be informed and that advice and guidance should be given by professionals. One consultant was concerned that the concept of choice was open to much interpretation: 'Ultimately, women should have the choice. But there are problems associated with unfettered choice. The implication of *Changing Childbirth* is that the women should choose *which* professional, *which* midwife. If you allow total choice, you may reduce the quality of care offered by the good practices to the lowest denominator... Home deliveries are not for those who make demands beyond those available at home – they should opt for hospital delivery. Otherwise the hospital and emergency staff are called out to them. This is to the disadvantage of other women and imperils the organisation of the hospital.'

A consultant in another hospital agreed that there should be choice but said: 'Home births should be discussed, but the safest place is in hospital, in my view. I assess and give my views, but ultimately, they decide. If there are physical reasons, my professional view will be to voice them, but ultimately it's their right and unfortunately the unborn baby has no legal right until after it is born. The unborn baby has no voice.'

Two consultants were against home births. One was quite adamant: 'It's anarchy. Dangerous! I'm totally concerned about the safety aspect. I'm yet to be convinced that there's anything wrong in women going into labour, coming into hospital for delivery and going home six hours later.'

Another was also concerned about safety: 'The infrastructure is just not in place to support large numbers of women like that, knowing that women can run into trouble having babies. If a proportion of women deliver at home, it is vital that they are at the lower end of the risk scale. There's no such thing as no risk. I firmly believe that hospital is the safest. As soon as they have the baby they can go home. But the process of labour and delivery is safer in hospital.'

It seemed doubtful in the course of these interviews whether the consultant obstetricians were aware of the extent to which the midwives in the midwifery group practices were encouraging women to consider home deliveries.

Women holding case notes

All the women under the care of all the consultant obstetricians held their own case notes throughout their pregnancies. All but one of the consultants were broadly in favour, mainly because the notes did not get lost and it was thought to have advantages in involving women in their own care and in having all the documentation readily available to all professionals in one place. However, one consultant thought that there were limits to its value: 'You can't put sensitive information into patients' notes. You don't record previous obstetric history – for example terminations – because the woman might not want her partner to know. And for similar reasons, important psycho-social factors are left out.'

One consultant thought it had no advantages: 'Flavour of the month. They are scruffy, dirty, too big for the handbag and get grease all over them.'

Aims of the midwifery group practices

The consultants held rather different views of what they understood the main aims of the midwifery group practices to be. Some used the same phrases, such as the provision of midwifery-led care, but interpreted them differently. For example, one consultant said the aim was: '...to explore the feasibility, acceptability and practical implications of running a midwifery-led service on perceived low-risk women.' He added that it could be argued that people who needed this approach most were the high risk women, for the continuity, trusting relationship, empathy and so on.

Another said the aims had not been spelt out clearly: 'The impression I get is that it is midwifery-led. I have no objection, provided that they are the "responsible" professional - that is, they have the ultimate responsibility. Are they indemnity insured?'

Others understood the main aims as providing community midwifery and to prevent hospital care or to provide an alternative to hospital care. Two of the consultants thought that the main aims included an increase in home births, which neither was happy about. Others mentioned the objective for as many women as possible to be delivered by a named midwife or one of a team, and to assess an appropriate method of delivering midwifery-based care to an inner London population on the basis of a midwifery group practice working in conjunction with patients, GPs and consultant obstetricians.

Although most of the consultants had heard of the midwifery group practices other than those using their own hospital, there was perhaps a surprising lack of knowledge among these consultant obstetricians that the SETRHA pilot had set up three midwifery group practices.

Care of consultants' patients by midwifery group practices

We were interested in the extent to which the women seen by the consultants during their pregnancy and/or delivery received midwifery care from any of the MGPs. In all cases, the local MGP gave care to patients seen by consultants, and one consultant had seen women cared for by the Deptford MGP.

We asked how the respective responsibilities of GP, group practice midwife and consultant obstetrician were agreed upon in these cases and, again, we asked specifically whether there were protocols which set out the relationships. There was little agreement.

One consultant said tersely: 'I don't know. There may be protocols. The midwives' attitude is – consultants stay out.' Another in the same hospital noted that there were no protocols: 'Not that I've seen. I'm not aware that this is spelt out even in the latest documentation. It astonishes me that it was set up without protocols.'

However, another consultant in the same hospital said that there had been a written protocol. There were problems, in his view, in establishing who had responsibility for the patient.

In the other hospital, there were said to be no protocols as such for deciding on the respective responsibilities of the various professionals in the case of the MGP. One consultant said: 'We have clear protocols for the hospital. As soon as the woman comes to me, the burden of responsibility falls to me. The midwife is not going to take responsibility. It's a question of accountability – who is accountable for what happens to the patient?' Another said: 'There has never been a problem between hospital doctors and midwives, or hospital doctors and GPs.'

Circumstances in which consultant would be lead professional

The question of when the consultant would be lead professional in cases where a woman received care from the MGP again brought up disagreement about the definition of the term 'lead professional'.

One consultant said: 'If you mean lead professional is the person that the woman would go to with queries – then that's the midwife. If you mean making the decisions with the patient – then that is me.'

Another consultant in the same hospital said that the consultant would be lead professional: '...when a woman chooses this option, or if there is a special reason or a complication, like a previous obstetric problem or a current medical problem. Or if midwifery care was booked and the complications arise requiring a transfer.'

Another consultant said he would be lead professional in cases of shared care: 'I share even if it's high risk – mostly shared care with the GP – very rarely with the midwife, but I've no aversion to doing this.' Others in the same hospital only took referrals from GPs, unless a woman was admitted for an emergency caesarean.

Most of the consultants felt that their role in the care of women attending the MGPs was no different from the role they usually took in the management of pregnancy and delivery. If they commented it was to say that this was mainly because they tended to see only high risk women or because they did not differentiate between the women.

Comparison of midwifery group practices with existing service provision

Three of the consultants thought that the services offered by the midwifery group practices had improved maternity services for women in their districts, one did not and one felt unable to comment.

Those who thought that the MGP services had improved maternity services mainly cited what they perceived to be increased satisfaction among the women using the service, but all of them qualified their remarks. One thought that it was impossible to assess outcomes since the numbers were too small. Another said that an audit on clinical and psychological outcomes would have to be carried out. One consultant was more concerned about the question of whether it could be more widely applied: 'It is operator dependent and the challenge is – can you get other midwives to do it? It's about the issue of change, but the other consideration is the needs of the midwives, who have responsibilities too. You still have your own kids that you have to get home to. Everyone seems to have forgotten that.'

Strengths and weaknesses of the midwifery group practices

The strengths of the midwifery group practices were seen by two consultants that they gave women more continuity of carer and three thought that they provided a 'patient-friendly' service. One said: 'The woman is booked at home and has a personalised midwife/pal to see her through the pregnancy.'

Another consultant thought that the main strength lay in 'reskilling and reestablishing the midwife's rightful role and place', while another thought that the close links between the MGP and the hospital and the mutual trust which had been established were particular strengths of the MGP.

The weaknesses identified by the consultants were interesting, in that none of the midwives themselves nor the GPs had come up with some of them, although our monitoring had indicated that some might be problems. One consultant who had plenty of praise for the MGP said: 'Inefficient practice is a concern – for example not seeing as many patients as they usefully could see in a given period of time. The issue is: the more freedom we give to midwives, the greater the risk of losing efficiency.'

Another who was equally enthusiastic about certain aspects of the MGP said: 'They have got carried away on the home birth issue. They have also forgotten that they are more committed than the run-of-the-mill midwife – and that affects the issue of extending it. There are a few limitations one might impose: there's a lot of home visiting which is unnecessary and they've gone overboard here. It's slightly worrying that the relationship between the midwife and the woman is described as friendship. For instance, I see a regular group of women and they trust me implicitly to do the right thing, but I wonder whether they would call me a friend. It may be different on a woman-to-woman basis.'

Another consultant were concerned that the midwives might be missing potential problems: 'You can have many normal pregnant women but when you look with a trained eye, they or the baby are actually at risk. It's wrong to by-pass the GP. I know these women are only pregnant – involving the uterus – but the GP is involved from top to tail. He should keep a finger on the pulse.'

And another consultant thought that screening in pregnancy was inadequately carried out by midwives and that they tended to refer problems too late, either to the GP or consultant, both because they lacked knowledge and experience and because they wanted to see the pilot project succeed.

Assessment of success

It was perhaps not surprising that the consultant obstetricians tended to put clinical outcomes at the top of their criteria for judging the success or otherwise of the midwifery group practices, although one consultant stressed that the numbers were too small for a proper assessment to be made. However, he emphasised that they should have 'acceptable safety'.

Most of the consultants added that client or patient satisfaction was an important criterion, although one disagreed, saying that patient satisfaction was 'a subjective thing'.

One consultant said that one of the main criteria was that they delivered good quality care at a cost acceptable to various commissioning authorities. 'It's not successful if they're nice but you can't afford them.' And another thought that costs and resources should also be taken into account in ensuring equitable distribution of services: 'You would have to assess the effect on the rest of the clinic. Does it take away too many resources from the hospital for this small number of women?'

The replicability of schemes of this nature was a criterion applied by another consultant: 'The ultimate test is being able to apply a project of that nature across a complete hospital or catchment area.'

It was perhaps not surprising that three of the five consultants felt unable to say how successful the MGP had been so far, according to their criteria. One thought it had been very successful and one thought it had been successful.

Among those who felt unable to comment on its success, one consultant said that it was impossible to assess because 'it's run by enthusiasts who want to make it work'. Another said: 'On maternal satisfaction, I would say very successful, because there have been few complaints. As for the midwives, it's difficult to say. Would they want to work that way for the rest of their careers? And on outcome measures – you can't make a valid comparison because it's a small group.'

Even among those who thought it successful, there were reservations: 'It's popular with patients and midwives, but not all midwives involved will want to take part. I believe the outcomes to be satisfactory, but costs are blurred and this is a real problem.'

What should have been done differently?

Looking back on the history of the midwifery group practice four of the consultant obstetricians thought that things should been done differently and one was not sure.

In Ashford, one consultant thought that the JACANES group should have stuck to the original protocol '...that is, providing care for low risk women. If they needed to expand, then JACANES II should have been the same, not a hybrid. It's valid to offer midwife-led care to high risk, but offer it as a second separate group.'

Another consultant thought that there should have been more consultation with hospital management and others, and was concerned about the drop-off in hospital antenatal clinic attendance which resulted in fewer training opportunities for junior doctors. And another was concerned about what he saw as a diminution in communications between professionals resulting from the pilot project.

One consultant thought the whole project should have been done at an earlier stage, while another was reluctant to pass any comments. He thought that pilot projects were useful in illustrating the potential benefits of a different approach, but reserved judgement on whether an independent evaluation would be able to assess the outcomes.

Replicability

Finally, considering all the doubts and reservations expressed by the consultant obstetricians, it was interesting to learn that all of them thought that the model of the midwifery group practices could be transferred to other districts in their present form. It was not, however surprising, that all the respondents imposed qualifications on their answers.

One said it could: '...in its original form of treating low risk women, and only if it fulfils the success criteria.' Another thought it could be transferred: '...but you must have keen midwives to undertake it, with a strict audit by a medical team, for example, one GP and one obstetrician.'

Others were more outspoken in their views: 'It could be transferred with modifications. I personally think ours is the most appropriate model for implementing *Changing Childbirth;* ours is the most realistic in terms of policy. Unfortunately, most of my colleagues are dinosaurs – not my local colleagues – and we all know what happened to dinosaurs...'

Chapter 9

Contracts, purchasing and funding arrangements

This chapter describes the funding arrangements for the three midwifery group practices (MGPs) and highlights both the similarities and the key differences. It looks at the purchaser and provider arrangements for each MGP and the nature of the service contracts. It also discusses the MGP budgets, and how each project used the £30,000 funding made available to them by SETRHA to assist with set-up costs and administrative support.

It is important at the outset to note that information about contracts, purchasing and funding arrangements was fragmented and required interviews with a range of providers and purchasers for each of the three MGPs. In each of the sites there was a level of uncertainty about the accuracy of some of the information provided, particularly regarding: the amount and source of funding for the MGPs; the entries in the MGP budgets; the specification of service contracts, and what these mean in practice. Frequently there were different interpretations of the data, not simply between purchasers and providers, but also between midwifery managers and finance/contract divisions where provider Trusts were involved.

LEWISHAM MATERNITY FOCUS

Purchaser and provider arrangements
The service provided by the Lewisham MGP (Lewisham Maternity Focus) was an integral part of the total obstetric and midwifery services provided by the Directorate of Women's Health Services at The Lewisham Hospital NHS Trust. The purchaser was Lambeth Southwark and Lewisham Health Commission (LSLHC), which, at the time of the monitoring, was made up of the Lambeth Southwark and Lewisham Family Health Services Authority and the South East London Health Authority. Obstetric and midwifery services were purchased from the Trust by the Acute Directorate at LSLHC.

The service contract with LSLHC did not show the MGP services separately from the total of obstetric and midwifery services purchased, and LSLHC did not monitor the MGP separately for contract purposes. LSLHC produced a service specification which applied to *all* of its contracts with provider institutions for maternity services. The service contract for 1995/96 referred to the *Changing Childbirth* report and stated that LSLHC was 'reviewing its purchases in the light of the report and producing a strategy for change. LSLHC wishes to encourage continued collaborative working with providers in this respect'. We understand, however, that while the health commission wanted the Trust to maintain and consolidate the progress made to date in the implementation of *Changing Childbirth,* in its 1996/97 purchasing intentions it did not envisage making additional funding available for this purpose.

Obstetric and midwifery services provided by Lewisham Hospital Trust were deliberately split into three categories for contract purposes. This enabled deliveries to be contracted separately, which was necessary because the Trust did not charge an average price per delivery across their total portfolio.

The price per delivery to Bromley, for example, was cheaper because women from that area delivering at Lewisham Hospital would receive most of their community midwifery care from Bromley midwives. The three purchasing categories are described below:

i) *Obstetric outpatients:* which referred to hospital outpatient/clinic based antenatal and postnatal attendances.

ii) *Obstetric delivery:* which covered everything that happened when a woman was in contact with the hospital on an inpatient basis, including antenatal, intrapartum and postnatal care. LSLHC purchased against deliveries and not finished consultant episodes (FCEs). It was estimated that one delivery on average was equivalent to 1.5 episodes of inpatient care per person. The 1995/96 contract indicated that LSLHC paid an average cost of approximately £1,372 per obstetric delivery.

iii) *Community midwifery:* which included the total cost of the community midwifery service purchased by LSLHC, and was made up of direct costs with no hospital overheads included. This cost included the MGP midwives who transferred into the MGP and were not additional to the establishment. The contract for 1995/96 showed a block figure of £600,000 for community midwifery. In addition, £180,000 was paid by LSLHC to the Trust in 1995/96 for additional midwives needed to keep the overall service up to standard.

MGP budget

The budget for Lewisham MGP covered midwives' salaries and on-call payments and expenses associated primarily with travel and use of telephones. No overtime payments were paid. Time was given in lieu and the team coordinated this amongst themselves. The majority of the funding came through the Directorate of Women's Health Services revenue budget, but some items of expenditure were met from regional funding.

Salaries

The biggest element of the budget was accounted for by the total cost of the salaries for the 5 grade G midwives and the 2 grade F midwives working in the practice. In 1994/95 actual expenditure on these midwives' salaries *(including* on-call payments) was around £226,000, a total which exceeded the estimated salaries budget for that period by around 19 per cent (approximately £37,000). The overspend arose from the actual level of on-call payments during this period.

Salary costs in 1995/96 were running at much the same rate as the costs in 1994/95. In April–September 1995/96 (up to the end of the monitoring period) approximately £92,500 was spent on midwife salaries *(excluding* on-call payments which were shown separately in 1995/96). In addition, the total for on-call costs for MGP midwives during this six-month period was in the region of £21,000, giving a total of £113,500. On this basis, on-call payments accounted for almost 19 per cent of total salary costs (basic salary costs plus on-call payments). This compares to a figure for the rest of the community midwives employed by Lewisham Hospital Trust of around 9 per cent for on-call payments as a percentage of total salary costs over the same period.

In Chapter 2 we demonstrated the ways in which the amount of on-call cover provided by individual midwives fluctuated and this was also evident in the on-call payments. The total amount of on-call payment claimed by each of the MGP midwives over the six-month period varied widely, from a minimum of around £2,000 up to the highest payment of approximately £4,500 (for one of the F grade midwives), with a mean total of approximately £3,050. The mean monthly on-call payment was around £500, but there were considerable monthly variations around the mean, not just between midwives but also for individual midwives over the six-month period.

Other expenditure

The estimated budget of approximately £16,000 for midwives' travel costs in 1994/95, which included lease car insurance, other lease car expenses and mileage claims, was underspent by around £4,000. This underspend on travel in the first year of the pilot was largely as a result of consideration being given to the amount of travelling each midwife was undertaking and the need to conduct visits in the most cost-effective pattern. In addition, the 1994/95 budget was based on the traditional community midwives' visits and work. For 1995/96 the budget was reduced and appears to have been adequate. In the first six months of the financial year 1995/96, MGP midwives' travel costs totalled approximately £6,400.

Telephone expenses for the midwives were mostly covered by the additional funds from the region (below) and not from within the Directorate. Approximately £2,000 was incurred in call charges by the 7 MGP midwives in 1994/95. Monthly figures supplied for telephone costs during April–September 1995 indicate that call charges were nearing £1,500 for this period, with considerable variation between calls attributed to individual midwives. We understand that from the middle of the year all midwives were urged to reduce their call charges and this was reflected in the monthly figures. Midwifery management estimated that a total of approximately £280-£300 per month was paid on cellphone expenses.

Funding from SETRHA

The £30,000 additional funding from SETRHA to assist with set-up costs and administrative support was a grant for two years. However, there seems to have been an issue locally, in both Lewisham and Ashford, as to how much, if any, could be carried over into the second year.

This additional money was used by the Lewisham MGP in a variety of ways, to cover items such as medical and surgical equipment, printing and stationery, office equipment and, as described above, cellphone expenses. An element was used for internal clinical audit sessions, given that clinical audit was outside the scope of the PSI evaluation. While the grant was drawn on to meet the costs of bank midwives for Lewisham Hospital, it was not used to pay for additional midwives for the MGP.

Overheads

The budget for the MGP covered only those direct costs funded from within the Directorate or from additional regional funding for the pilot. It did not, therefore, include all the costs that had to be reflected in the full price of the service charged to LSLHC. In particular, it did not include overheads – for example, recharges of heating, lighting, general management and so on – that had to be taken into account in the overall pricing structure and included in contract negotiations. These additional costs associated with running the MGP were charged on to the purchaser within the main contract for midwifery and obstetric services.

JACANES MIDWIFERY GROUP PRACTICE

Purchaser and provider arrangements

The service provided by the JACANES midwifery group practice in Ashford was part of the obstetric and midwifery services purchased by East Kent Health Authority (EKHA) from the Obstetrics and Gynaecology Division (William Harvey Hospital) of South Kent Hospitals NHS Trust.

The service contract between the Trust and EKHA did not separately identify the MGP from other community midwifery services. The contract was split into three categories for purchasing purposes and these are described below:

i) *Obstetric inpatients:* were purchased on a *finished consultant episode (FCE)* basis, and not deliveries as was the case in Lewisham. The 1995/96 contract allowed for 4,827 FCEs at a unit cost of £858. An FCE included deliveries and other inpatient stays involving the consultant. Hence FCEs did not equal the number of births.

ii) *Obstetric outpatients:* were purchased on a hospital outpatient attendance basis, usually at consultant clinics. The 1995/96 contract allowed for a total of £11,399 (initial and follow-up attendances), with a unit price of £45.

iii) *Community midwifery:* this element of the contract was less well developed than the calculations for obstetrics and there were differences in the interpretation put on the figures in the contract by the Trust and by EKHA. The contract was based around indicative contacts, domiciliary visits and sessions and was based on what the midwives recorded the year before. Community midwifery was purchased as a block contract, i.e. the Trust got £930,354 regardless of actual activity.

As part of the 1995/96 Contract for Health Care Services EKHA produced a service description and service objectives which were being revised in the light of *Changing Childbirth.*

MGP budget

The budget for the JACANES MGP covered midwives' salaries and on-call payments and expenses associated primarily with travel and use of telephones. No overtime payments were paid. Instead, time was taken in lieu by the midwives when their work commitments allowed. The majority of the funding came through the revenue budget for the Obstetrics and Gynaecology Division, but some items of expenditure were met from regional funding.

Salaries

For 1994/95 the annual cost of salaries for the JACANES I midwives (initially 4 grade Gs and 2 grade Fs) was approximately £130,500. This excluded around £15,000 which appeared in the budget for 1994/95 and which can be attributed to the salaries of the JACANES II midwives (see below). In addition, the total of on-call payments paid to the midwives during this period for rostered on-call amounted to around £3,100. This can be attributed primarily to one midwife being paid for on-call duty per night. On this basis on-call payments amounted to around 2.5 per cent of total costs (basic salary plus on-call payments). JACANES on-call cost were considerably less than those for the Lewisham MGP, reflecting the different on-call staffing arrangements and significantly lower level of on-call cover for JACANES described in Chapter 2 and Appendix B.

As we have explained, the caseload carried by JACANES I soon became excessive and detrimental to the aims of the MGP. It was decided that a second MGP was required to share the load, and in early 1995 EKHA provided around £90,000 additional (non-recurrent) funding to meet the cost of employing three additional midwives for this purpose. In addition, two other midwives were transferred from the current hospital staffing into JACANES II.

Since the establishment of JACANES II the budget figures for the two MGPs have been combined for accounting purposes. It has not been possible, therefore, to isolate the costs for JACANES I since February 1995. We cannot simply divide the figures by the number of midwives in the two MGPs because JACANES I and JACANES II have different case-mixes. To have separated out the figures would have involved considerable retrospective recoding work, and, given our focus on the resources used rather than actual costs, we did not feel justified in placing this extra burden on the accounting staff.

In addition to the midwives' salaries, administrative support was provided to the MGP on a part-time basis (8 hours a week) by one of the nursing auxiliaries. For a full year this support would have cost around £1,800.

Other expenditure

Other expenditure incurred by the MGP in 1994/95 was mostly on travel, telephones and equipment as described below. Actual expenditure for February and March 1995 included the costs incurred by the JACANES II midwives and this contributed to any variances which occurred between the estimated budget and actual expenditure for 1994/5.

- *Travel:* (approximately £17,000), mostly mileage allowances, but also including some lease car charges and insurance. There was a variance of around £4,000 between the projected budget and the actual spend. The caseload was larger than expected and this in turn would have generated more travel costs.

- *Telephone:* (approximately £2,300), including all mobile telephone costs and pagers.

- *Equipment:* (approximately £7,250), covering set-up equipment for the new midwives who had not worked in the community before.

Funding from region

The £30,000 made available by SETRHA was used primarily for administrative support for the pilot scheme. For example, computer hardware and software were bought to support the internal clinical audit. Some of the grant also went on the cost of telephones, and on the rental of a hall for drop-in sessions.

Overheads

As with the Lewisham project the JACANES budget covered only those costs which were controlled by the midwifery manager. There was cross-subsidisation between mainstream services and the MGP as illustrated by the following costs which were excluded from the MGP budget statement:

- supplies used from the hospital;

- overheads for heating, lighting and so on;

- around one fifth of the cost of the midwifery manager (included in the midwifery management support budget);

- an element for the clinical director, business manager, support staff.

These overheads had to be reflected in the contract prices paid by EKHA for obstetric and midwifery services.

DEPTFORD MIDWIFERY GROUP PRACTICE

Purchaser and provider arrangements

The Deptford MGP was a community based project offering a self-managed midwifery service. Whereas the midwives in Lewisham and JACANES were employed by their respective Hospital Trusts, the MGP midwives were self-employed.

The midwifery services provided by the Deptford MGP were purchased primarily by Lambeth Southwark and Lewisham Health Commission (LSLHC). Whereas the *Acute Directorate* at LSLHC was responsible for contracting with Lewisham Hospital for services which included the Lewisham MGP, the *Primary Care Directorate* was responsible at the time of writing this report for contracting with the Deptford MGP using Tomlinson money (Primary Care Development Fund).

The MGP had to demonstrate that it was a service providing intensive care for women with special needs to justify using Tomlinson money as a source of funding, and this requirement was reflected in the contract in terms of target groups and quotas to be met. The MGP aimed to target certain groups who were often denied choice, might require intensive care and support, or who had particular socio-economic factors in their lives that had been identified as placing their babies more at risk. The access criteria set in the contract with LSLHC for 1995 were tighter than those for 1994. Under the 1995/96 contract at least 50 per cent of all services were reserved for residents of Deptford. The MGP had to reserve a quota of 80 per cent, up from 75 per cent, for the target groups, and the specification for 'women with mental health difficulties' was tightened.

The contract with LSLHC was let in phases. The original agreement for the provision of midwifery services covered the period 1 April 1994 to 31 March 1995 and was for 50 episodes of care. Under this contract LSLHC agreed that payment for the service would be made in the form of two block payments, each of £25,000, in May and September. Payments were subject to the satisfactory provision of information required for monitoring and review, including demonstration that the terms of the contract were being fulfilled. In the event, LSLHC eventually funded over-performance on the contract up to 20 episodes.

The second agreement for 1995/96 was for 80 episodes of care in the first instance. In a separate protocol, provision was made for an additional 50 episodes in August 1995, providing the MGP satisfied LSLHC that negotiations on sub-contracting with acute unit(s) were well advanced. This linked to the fact that the Primary Care Directorate could not continue funding the service using development money. At the time of writing, if the MGP was to continue, alternative funding arrangements would need to be established and one option was for the MGP to secure a sub-contract arrangement with one or more acute units.

The Deptford MGP was on the catchment area boundary of Lewisham and Greenwich, and Greenwich and Bexley (G&B) Health Authority also purchased midwifery services from the MGP. Using Tomlinson money they purchased the service by means of two annual grants, covering 20 episodes of care in 1994/5 and 22 episodes in 1995/6, with the possibility of 12 further episodes over and above the second contract.

In practice there were a number of problems and misunderstandings concerning this MGP's funding, particularly in the initial year. One issue was that it became apparent that there was a gap between the number of episodes to be purchased by the Health Commissions, and the number of bookings (200 women) that the MGP were expected to reach to fulfil the requirements of their bid and the evaluation.

An associated complication was that before the pilot started in April 1994 the midwives were already caring for a group of around 70 women who had previously booked as self-financing clients and therefore did not receive all their care under the terms of the pilot MGP (see Chapter 3 and Appendix C). Nonetheless, the MGP transferred some of the funding which LSLHC had intended for new clients, booked from April 1994, to cover the cost of providing the service to this existing group of women. This transfer meant that the MGP quickly exceeded the number of women covered under the service agreement, and that some of these women had been booked before the start date covered by the agreement.

In reviewing the contract it was unclear to LSLHC whether the MGP had met the terms of the contract to see mostly under-privileged women, and the payment of the second instalment of funding due in September 1994 became uncertain. This in turn led to the midwives ceasing to book women after 15 August 1994 and to their seeking funds from other sources. A bid for private sector funding was unsuccessful and negotiations were started to operate on a sub-contract basis with an acute unit. Further discussions with LSL and G&B Health Commissions eventually resulted in the Health Commissions making full payment under the initial contracts and purchasing the additional episodes of care described above, thus enabling the MGP to budget for approximately 150 episodes of care in 1995/96.

Episode of care

LSL and G&B Health Commissions purchased services from the Deptford MGP on the basis of 'an episode of midwifery care covering the period from initial booking up to and including the postnatal period'. The postnatal period referred to the period of time from birth and up to 28 days after birth. This definition of an episode of care was quite different from the contracting arrangements which applied to the Lewisham and JACANES MGPs. The decision to purchase care from Deptford MGP on this basis was a deliberate choice by LSLHC because they wanted to test out an intensive service for clients with special needs.

Price

The midwives reported that in the first year they had no sound benchmark for their costs except those encountered as independent midwives. The original price per episode of care to LSLHC and G&B Health Commission was £1,000. This was increased to £1,100 in the second year to reflect more accurately their costs and overheads, and to enable the MGP to fulfil the requirements of the evaluation.

The purchase price did not include hospital charges or ambulance costs associated with the women using the Deptford MGP which LSLHC would, for example, pay for under their main acute contracts for obstetrics and midwifery care. However, when a woman using the Deptford MGP attended hospital for a consultation or for a delivery her Deptford midwife would aim to accompany her. The main hospital costs excluded from the price were:

- ultrasound
- laboratory facilities
- referral to obstetrician, paediatrician, haematologist etc.
- elective/emergency hospital delivery.

It was up to the midwives to negotiate service agreements with individual hospitals.

LSLHC considered that there was a value-added dimension to the cost of the services obtained from Deptford MGP. The pregnancy testing service, antenatal groups, health advice, and interpreters could be accessed by any women in the area, and not just by those who were counted among the episodes of care paid for by the Health Commission.

MGP budget

The budget and accounts for the Deptford MGP give details of the group's income and expenditure.

Income

Income was obtained mainly through NHS contracts with LSLHC and G&B Health Commission to provide midwifery services. This was topped up with the funding from SETRHA and from donations.

Salaries

Deptford MGP midwives considered themselves to be ungraded and to have no set hours. As a benchmark their salaries were based on the equivalent of a community midwife grade G, with the top increment including London Weighting, who would then receive additional payments for own car use, unsociable hours, weekend, on-call and overtime payments. Deptford's fee structure was also intended to take into account the fact that they were self-managing.

On this basis, in their bid to operate as a pilot project the MGP midwives estimated that in their first year of operation they would each draw a fee of £25,000. Individual midwives were expected to cover their own travel/car expenses (around £2,000 per annum), provide capital midwifery equipment (worth around £1,000) and cover additional expenses (such as telephone at home, indemnity insurance) estimated at between £5,000 and £10,000. In addition they costed around £11,200 for a part-time administrator.

In the event, the difficulties described above in implementing their funding arrangement with LSLHC and G&B Health Commission, and the confusion over bookings, resulted in their actual drawings in 1994/95 being limited to approximately half-pay.

In their business plan for 1995/96 the midwives' fee was projected at £27,000 per annum pro rata for a full caseload. The estimated budget demonstrated that the project needed funding for the projected 150 episodes of care in order to be financially viable. In addition to the midwives' fees, other staffing costs included the practice manager and the women's health resource coordinator who each worked 3 full days (21 hours) per week. They expected to draw pro rata earnings of approximately £19,000, based on social work grading scale 3.

Indemnity insurance

The LSLHC contract stipulated that the self-employed midwives would have to cover their own indemnity insurance. This was a problem for the MGP since the Royal College of Midwives withdrew insurance cover for independent midwives as part of their membership package. It was estimated that insurance companies would charge premiums comparable to those for obstetricians – i.e. in the region of £7,000 per year – and this would increase the MGP's prices unacceptably. In the event indemnity insurance cost around £5,000 per midwife and LSLHC assisted Deptford with a grant towards the bill; the rest had to be borne by the practice.

Other expenditure

The income and expenditure account for 1994/95 show that the expenses of the MGP (over and above staffing costs) totalled around £12,000. This included items such as room hire; printing, postage and stationery; consultancy; subscriptions; telephone; repairs and maintenance; accountancy; sundries; and depreciation.

In the business plan for 1995/6 the main projected items of expenditure for the MGP (based on 150 episodes of care) included:

- *Premises costs:* (approximately £10,000), at the Albany Centre where heating and lighting were included in the rent .

- *Running costs:* (approximately £6,150), which included telephone, office equipment, computer and printer, stationery, photocopying, stamps and meeting facilities.

- *Midwifery supplies:* (approximately £6,000), which covered costs such as message pagers, disposable equipment, Entonox cylinder hire/refills, maintenance of equipment and pregnancy testing kits.

- *Service provision:* (approximately £5,250), which included the hire of rooms and the use of a creche for afternoon antenatal and postnatal groups, the printing of leaflets and the freelance use of interpreters.

- *Professional fees:* (approximately £2,600), which covered management consultants, group facilitators, computer training, accountancy and solicitors' costs.

- *Library costs and subscriptions to journals* (approximately £1,200).

Funding from SETRHA

The £30,000 pump priming grant from SETRHA was budgeted to cover consultancy costs, computer equipment and set costs associated with practice staff and office expenses. In practice, some of this money was drawn on in the initial stages of the pilot, along with donations, to keep the MGP afloat while contractual issues were negotiated with purchasers.

Issues arising

The above account of the purchasing and funding arrangements for the three MGPs generates a number of issues which have a bearing on what is feasible in terms of further analysis about costs and cost-effectiveness and what conclusions can be drawn.

In particular the following points are significant:

- in general, detailed comparisons between the costs of the three MGPs are inappropriate because the cost bases were quite different;

- each of three MGPs operated with a quite different definition and pricing structure for an episode of care;

- the apparent 'cost-effectiveness' of the service depended partly on how the overheads were apportioned, and the methods of apportionment and opportunities for cross-subsidisation differed considerably between the MGPs. Cross-subsidisation and hidden overheads could occur in relation to the Lewisham and JACANES MGPs, where the MGP was integral to the total obstetric and midwifery services provided by the respective Trusts. This was not the case with the Deptford MGP, which was effectively a business partnership and had to produce full income and expenditure accounts;

- duplication of costs might have occurred where women crossed boundaries. They might also have arisen where women transferred between the MGPs. The amount of duplication would have depended on the charging policies of the providers involved and how they defined and contracted for an episode of care. Duplication could also have arisen between the MGPs and General Practice item of service payments for maternity care.

Different funding practices which were not transparent, along with difficulties in obtaining good quality, reliable financial data have limited what was achievable in terms of reporting on the costs and cost-effectiveness of the MGPs. Wherever possible we have described and commented on the costs involved, but, given the unavailability or inaccuracy of much of the existing cost data, we considered it more useful in this report to concentrate on the level and type of resources required to operate and sustain the midwifery group practices as developed in each of the three pilot sites. This type of analysis and insight will be more meaningful to other local purchasers and providers in planning for the future of midwifery care.

Chapter 10

Discussion of findings

This report has examined a very broad range of issues which have been raised through the setting up of three midwifery group practice pilot projects by South East Thames Regional Health Authority (SETRHA) in 1993. We have described in detail the monitoring and evaluation of these pilot projects carried out by Policy Studies Institute over the 18-month period from 1 April 1993 to 30 September 1995. In this discussion of findings, we draw together the main threads of our research, which was conducted using a variety of methods, and explore the implications for practice and policy of the models of working established by the three midwifery group practices.

It should be stressed from the outset that our aim is to draw out the lessons that can be learnt from the experience of all those involved in the pilot projects. Demonstration projects of this kind, set up with limited funding for a limited time period, with little lead-in time, usually with staff who have not worked together before, with new methods of management and practice, with high expectations and little experience of managing change, can expect to experience multiple problems (for example, see Allen, 1991; Williams and Allen, 1989). Those working in such projects have been described as 'heroic pioneers', with high levels of dedication and a determination to succeed in proving that their innovative practices can be replicated and should be widely adopted elsewhere. This chapter will underline how true this was of the staff in the three pilot midwifery group practices, but it will also highlight how difficult it is, not only to implement changes in working practices in isolation from mainstream service provision, but also to demonstrate success over the short-term, particularly in the absence of an adequate planning period.

It should be accepted that there are fundamental differences between evaluating demonstration projects and carrying out a controlled trial, and that they demand different approaches. One of the main aims of setting up demonstration projects is to see what can be learnt from the experience of developing practice, rather than demonstrating in fine detail the areas of similarities and differences with a control group. In this evaluation we have drawn very little on evidence from comparative sources, mainly because of the time and resource constraints under which we, like the pilot projects themselves, were operating. But we hope that through this chapter we will identify the areas for further work and analysis which could usefully be carried out.

The context

The pilot projects were set up by SETRHA as a result of the considerable pressures to change maternity services which had been building up over some years, culminating in *Changing Childbirth,* the report of the Expert Maternity Group chaired by Baroness Cumberlege (Department of Health, 1993). We have already seen that the main findings of this report were that maternity services should be designed to allow women more control over their care, should offer choice of treatment, lead professional and place of delivery, and should aim to provide greater continuity of care and carer.

Following the publication of the House of Commons Health Select Committee's Second Report on Maternity Services (1992), SETRHA sponsored a Consensus Conference on *Maternity Services for the Future* (SETRHA, 1992), which called for the establishment of pilot schemes for autonomous midwifery group practices. We have described in Chapter 1 the hypothesis put forward by SETRHA that the pilot projects would provide high quality and cost-effective services for women and their families, who would exhibit increased satisfaction with the service. This hypothesis was based on assumptions that the development of such midwifery group practices would improve continuity of care and carer; would facilitate direct access to midwives; would give women greater choice of carer through strengthening the role of midwives; would improve the self-esteem of midwives; would reduce duplication of services; would clarify roles and responsibilities of all practitioners and professionals involved; and would not reduce safety.

Policy Studies Institute's role was to examine the extent to which these assumptions were well-founded, to see to what extent the outcomes of the evaluation were related to the implementation of practice based on these assumptions, and to provide an overall evaluation with special attention to costs, role clarification of practitioners, access to midwives, improvements in the continuity of care and choice available for women, and client satisfaction.

The structure and organisation of the midwifery group practices

The report has described in considerable detail the structure and organisation of the midwifery group practices, both within the text and in the Appendices. The complexities of organising and managing 'autonomous' group practices of professionals cannot be underestimated, and one of the clear messages from this evaluation is that the potential demands on the midwives in operating a new system must be properly assessed before anyone embarks upon putting it into practice. There is no substitute for careful planning if resources are to be managed in the most efficient and effective way and if practitioners are not to suffer from overload.

Many of the problems encountered by the midwives in all three group practices could have been prevented, or at least circumvented, by more realistic appraisals of the actual numbers of women for whom they would be caring, the ways in which their duty rota and on-call arrangements would work in practice, the extent to which they could actually ensure the continuity of carer for which they aimed, and the impact on their own personal lives in attempting to provide a coverage of considerably greater intensity than was feasible either for themselves in the long-term or, more important, was capable of being replicated or 'rolled out' more generally. The projects and their evaluation have played a valuable role in highlighting these critical factors and providing a sounder basis on which to approach future planning.

There can be little doubt, in assessing the data collected for this evaluation, that many of the real resource implications of providing services of the type provided by the midwifery group practices were hidden, not only from the researchers, but also from the managers, often because they were not properly recognised or acknowledged by the midwives themselves. The constant stress on 'informal' or 'flexible' arrangements in the provision of care to women on midwives' individual caseloads, over and above the rota or on-call duties of the midwives, made the task of assessing the real workload of the midwives almost impossible. But, more important, it also made a realistic appraisal of cost-effectiveness even more difficult. We will look further at the difficulties in making any conclusive statements about costs, but it should be borne in mind throughout this discussion of findings that the true resource implications of these models of practice were almost as difficult to assess definitively as the real costs involved.

Setting up and the initial stages

What were the main problems in setting up and organising the midwifery group practices? The three pilot projects were very different from one another, but there can be no doubt that the Deptford practice had particular problems which were unique to them as a group of independent midwives essentially operating outside the National Health Service, at least to begin with. Unlike the other two projects they had no ready referral source from GP practices, they had no inbuilt links with specific hospitals and they had no management and organisational back-up.

Not least, because they had no historically sound referral base, they were able to establish only limited guaranteed funding from local health commissions, geared to a requirement that they should deliver care to a strictly targeted group of women with specified health and social problems quite different from those of most women to whom the individual midwives in the group had previously provided care. Although the Deptford midwives said that they had operated a 'Robin Hood' approach in their previous practice, the analysis of the socio-demographic characteristics of the women they brought with them into the monitoring period shows clearly that most were professional or middle-class women, completely unlike the group for whom they were required to provide services under the contractual arrangement with the commissioning agencies during the monitoring period.

The biggest problem for the Deptford practice was therefore getting started and maintaining a service by attracting new clients. Their funding initially mainly went to support existing clients, which may not have been the most appropriate way of using the resources, and they had great difficulties in attracting new referrals. Much of their time and energy in the first few months was spent trying to solve all the problems involved in setting up a small business, which distracted them from their aim of delivering high quality midwifery care. The fact that they were able to sustain a high level of midwifery practice which women found satisfactory was undoubtedly related to the fact that they had relatively few women on their books. There must be doubts about whether they could have sustained the type and level of care they offered if they had had more clients. Even at the end of the monitoring period, they were running well below the capacity expected of the midwifery group practices. A true evaluation of the model offered by the Deptford midwifery group practice was not possible during the monitoring period, since they never operated at anything approaching full capacity, in terms of booking, antenatal care or deliveries.

The other two midwifery group practices in Lewisham and Ashford were much more similar in terms of history and structure and comparisons between them were easier to make. It was also possible to assess them more appropriately in terms of mainstream maternity services, and to draw some conclusions on whether and how the models of services they provided were replicable elsewhere.

The main problem in Ashford was that the midwives were essentially operating a double caseload for at least the first nine or ten months of the monitoring period. Although their bid stated that they would only provide full continuity of care and carer as lead professional for around 200 women with uncomplicated pregnancies, including delivery, they also envisaged providing some antenatal and postnatal care to women with complicated pregnancies, working in conjunction with the GP or consultant obstetrician. In the event, what happened was that the midwives operated on a basis of offering choice to a high proportion of the women with whom they came into contact, including high risk women. Their workload of antenatal and postnatal care exploded, so that the actual numbers of women they were caring for reached some 500 a year, as opposed to the 200 for which their infrastructure and organisation was designed.

Essentially, the Ashford midwives did not adhere to the protocol they had established before the projects started for directing women to midwifery group practice, GP or consultant-led care. Choice was offered to all-comers, women who had had previous care from particular midwives were treated 'flexibly' and the problem was only solved by introducing another group of midwives, JACANES II, to care for high-risk women nearly a year after the start of the monitoring period, thus virtually doubling the number of midwifery staff covering the caseload which had been handled by the original midwifery group practice for a considerable part of the monitoring period.

In Lewisham, continuing problems also related to overload, and throughout the monitoring period it was clear that the midwifery group practice was offering care to greater numbers of women than it had planned for. One of the interesting issues which arose in both Ashford and Lewisham related to the traditional manner in which midwifery terminology obscures the actual workload of midwives. The use of the word caseload is not helpful in assessing the true workload of midwives, and in all three midwifery group practices there appeared to be a reluctance to acknowledge the fact that the number of bookings in a year does not equal the number of deliveries, and that there may be a considerable workload involved in providing booking and antenatal care to women who, for one reason or another, are not delivered by the midwives. In Lewisham this was related not only to women who moved or who had miscarriages but also to women who delivered in other local hospitals. Counting deliveries alone does not give a true indication of workload. A careful analysis is also necessary in establishing the true cost of midwifery care, including all antenatal, intrapartum and postnatal care.

Although the evaluators drew attention to the continuing high numbers of women being cared for in Lewisham, no action was taken to reduce numbers during the monitoring period. There were doubts about the longer-term sustainability of the workload of the midwives but staffing levels prevented any further recruitment to the midwifery group practice until after the end of the monitoring period. As we have seen in the report, they changed some of their actual practice over the monitoring period in order to reduce the undoubted fatigue from which most suffered, with the acknowledgement that this was not enough.

Continuity of care and carer
The provision of continuity of care and carer in maternity services were key recommendations of *Changing Childbirth*. It was argued that this was what women wanted and that it could lead both to an improved quality of care and to greater job satisfaction for midwives. We were interested in

assessing to what extent the midwifery group practices achieved this aim and we set out to examine the constraints, both organisational or in resource terms, to providing such continuity. We also attempted to assess whether any particular model was more likely to ensure the goal of continuity, and whether it could only be achieved with more limited numbers of women or at greater personal or financial cost than had been envisaged when these pilot projects were set up.

All three of the midwifery group practices felt that they achieved a high degree of continuity of care and carer, and the statistical evidence and the evidence from the women confirms that this was certainly true in Lewisham and Deptford. In Ashford, the situation was complicated by the fact that the midwives could not have hoped to provide continuity of care or carer for the vastly inflated number of women for whom they were providing care during the first year of monitoring. However, we established evidence that they were able to provide continuity of care for the 200 low risk women envisaged in their protocol.

There were interesting developments over the monitoring period in how the Lewisham and Ashford practices organised the way in which they achieved continuity of care. Initially it was seen vital for midwives to have their own caseloads and for women to have named midwives. These were seen as important characteristics of midwifery group practices and fundamental to achieving continuity of care. However, as the midwives established trust among themselves and recognised that they had shared goals in achieving their aims, the emphasis on individual caseloads began to shift and by the end of the monitoring period, midwives began to distinguish between continuity of care and continuity of carer, commenting that continuity of care could be achieved without total continuity of carer.

There were also indications that some midwives recognised that too much emphasis on continuity of carer carried the risk of creating too great a dependency in the relationship between midwife and client. This recognition was certainly borne out in comments made by the women we interviewed, some of whom graphically illustrated the dependent relationships they had formed with their midwives. This has important implications, not only in preventing the formation of good relationships with other key professionals such as GPs, who, as we have seen, often felt totally excluded during the antenatal period, but also in the engendering of dependent relationships with midwives who could neither sustain the relationship nor, perhaps, were the best-equipped to do so. For many years, one of the important criticisms of the plethora of professional workers visiting people with multiple problems has been the extent to which lack of liaison and communication can lead to the fostering of dependent relationships with one professional when other professionals may be trying to establish independence. Midwives are not psychiatrists, doctors or social workers, and professional parameters of competence and expertise should be recognised and acknowledged by all professionals.

The women interviewed for this study were mainly delighted with the continuity of care and carer provided by the midwifery group practices, and many made comparisons with previous pregnancies in which they saw different professionals each time or were treated by a number of different professionals on each occasion. However, as we have observed throughout this report, many of the comments made by women about their previous maternity care relate more to inadequacies in the organisation of hospital or community practice rather than to the need for a completely innovative system of working with all the potential resource implications. Many of the criticisms we heard from women of previous care described poor practice, poor interpersonal skills on the part of staff and poor organisation. It should not be assumed that continuity of care and carer will solve problems like these. It could be argued that the key factor is the quality of the care and carer rather than its continuity alone. Continuous care from a poor carer may be even more unsatisfactory than care from a variety of professionals.

Therefore in assessing the success of the midwifery group practices in providing continuity of care and carer, it is important to disentangle the different elements involved. The move over the monitoring period by both the Lewisham and Ashford midwifery group practices towards sharing the workload underlined the difficulties in resource and personal terms of providing guaranteed intrapartum care by the named midwife. It was also clear that women were not as concerned about continuity of carer throughout as many of the midwives were. Women laid more stress on the quality of the care which they received from the midwifery group practices in general and were usually happy to receive care from any member of the team.

The resource implications of providing continuity of care were difficult to establish fully. In Deptford, where midwives worked essentially with a single caseload but in partnership with one other midwife, the potential resource implications were very high, in that midwives were always on-call for their own women. This constant 24-hour cover requirement on all midwives on a continuous basis helped to create tension and overload. It was not sustainable for all the midwives, and was partly responsible for the changing composition of the group during the monitoring period. It was also clear that it would not have been sustainable for the group working at the capacity envisaged in the protocol.

In Ashford, it was clearly impossible for the midwives to provide continuity for their full caseload, but we have seen that they appeared to be able to manage it for 200 women, with the proviso that they would not be able to guarantee the presence of the named midwife at delivery, although they attempted to provide cover for women on their own caseloads as well as providing on-call cover on a rota basis.

In Lewisham, the named midwife was present at a very high proportion of deliveries, but there were resource implications in the way in which this was made possible, some of which were apparent, but many of which were hidden. The system of having two midwives on-call 24 hours as cover, as opposed to one midwife on day and one on night cover in Ashford, was clearly more expensive, but the sometimes hidden costs by which midwives also provided intrapartum care for their own caseload should be taken into account when assessing the overall resource implications, not only in terms of cost, but also in terms of personal overload on midwives.

It should be noted that a model where midwives work in partnership and provide continuous cover for their own caseloads is already in operation within the NHS. Not surprisingly the model has been introduced with an important modification on that operating in Deptford: midwives are paid an annual negotiated rate for providing on-call cover.

Direct access to midwives

Direct access to midwives without having to go through a referral route has been recommended and one of the assumptions of SETRHA in setting up these pilot projects was that direct access to midwives would be facilitated if the maternity services were community centred. However, there are various questions which arise concerning direct access to midwives. For example, is direct access to midwives necessarily always in the best interests of all women? What are the implications of direct access to midwives in terms of offering greater choice of care and carer? What are the implications of direct access to midwives in ensuring liaison and good relationships between the various professionals involved in the provision of maternity care? And, in any case, is direct access to midwives an important issue for women? Is it what they want?

It appeared that direct access to midwives was not an important issue for women in either Lewisham or Ashford. Women assumed that the normal first point of contact in pregnancy was to go to their GP for confirmation of pregnancy and to discuss options. Most women saw their GP first, and direct access to midwives occurred mainly on an ad hoc basis, sometimes when receptionists gave positive pregnancy test results and asked if women wanted to see the midwives and sometimes when women already knew midwives from previous pregnancies.

There was little evidence that women in Lewisham and Ashford wanted direct access to midwives and plenty of evidence that they regarded it as natural to see their GPs. Indeed, it was clear from our interviews that some women were rather surprised that their GPs appeared diffident about discussing their pregnancies and sent them to the midwives. Instead of feeling that they had been offered a choice of care and carer by the GPs, many women assumed that midwifery-led care was the only care available. There were indications that, as a result, some women felt that it was not appropriate for them to consult their GPs about their maternity care and, in some cases, felt rather let down by their GPs.

There can be little doubt that there was considerable confusion among both women and GPs about how the midwifery group practices would operate in terms of choice of care and carer. As our interviews with the GPs in the 'host practices' showed, many GPs felt sidelined and left out by the introduction of the midwifery group practices. They were unclear about how and by whom the women would be presented with a choice of care and carer, but most had assumed that they themselves would still be involved in the care of their patients during pregnancy, birth and the post-natal period. It only became clear to them as the monitoring period progressed that they were seeing very few pregnant women, which resulted in their dissatisfaction with the system which has been described in detail in the report and will be discussed further below. It must have been apparent that increased direct access to midwives would not improve relationships between midwives and GPs unless there were clear protocols for liaison and collaboration which were agreed and adhered to.

Direct access to midwives was clearly more of an issue for the Deptford midwives who had no regular referral source. The fact that women could come directly to them without going through a referral process was a key factor in their bid for funding in the SETRHA initiative. There can be no doubt that the success of independent midwives in attracting a faithful clientele indicates that there are women for whom direct access to a midwife is important, although other factors in the care they are given may be more important to them.

The Deptford midwives set up a shopfront walk-in service in a small community centre which offered pregnancy testing and counselling as well as midwifery care. There were indications that it brought in women who were dissatisfied for one reason or another with their existing pregnancy care. We have seen that a high proportion of the Deptford cases were women who had received at least some of their antenatal care elsewhere and that a significant proportion transferred at a very late stage in their pregnancy to the Deptford practice. It could be argued that direct access to midwives by vulnerable and disadvantaged women raises issues of a more complex nature than simply direct access.

We have already referred to the potential dangers of conflicting and confusing messages being given to women already receiving care from a number of agencies and professionals. The lack of liaison between professionals which may ensue from pursuing a policy of direct access to midwives as a matter of prime importance may be inappropriate in many cases. It may mean that important general health information relating to women is not available to midwives. It may also mean that, if women transfer at a late stage in their pregnancy to directly accessed midwives, important antenatal information may not be available.

Greater choice for women through strengthening role of midwives

One of the assumptions of SETRHA in setting up the pilot projects was that women would be given greater choice through strengthening the role of midwives in group practices. There are a number of areas in maternity care in which issues of choice may arise. We have already touched on choice of care and choice of carer. There is also the question of choice of home birth or hospital birth. There are also issues surrounding pain control in labour and delivery, and the type of delivery. And, not least, there are issues around the location, frequency, timing and length of ante-natal consultations and similar issues around postnatal consultations. In addition, it should be remembered that in recommending greater choice for women, there has also been an assumption that women should be offered the option to change their minds.

In examining the question of choice, there are many areas which need to be examined in detail. We were interested in looking at how and by whom choices were presented to women, the selection of women for whom choices were appropriate, the question of 'informed' choice, and whether or not real options were presented at all. We asked specific questions of our respondents about these areas, but they often raised many issues regarding the interpretation of the word 'choice', the question of whether choice should be offered at all in certain circumstances, for example those affecting the safety of the woman or her baby, the question of what happens when the choice of a woman conflicts with the clinical judgement of professionals, and, not least, the general question of the extent to which the choices of users of services can be met when resources are finite and services must be rationed. Some of these issues are common to a whole range of services, but others are specific to maternity services.

We looked at the issue of *choice of carer* in pregnancy, and found that there was considerable confusion among the various groups of interested parties whom we interviewed. It was quite clear from our interviews with women in Lewisham and Ashford that many of them did not understand, either from their consultations with GPs or with midwives, that they might have a choice of carer. Since these two midwifery group practices were based in GP practices with the purpose of offering choice of carer or 'lead professional', this finding was rather surprising. It appeared that the lack of clear protocols in both areas relating to the offering of choice to women resulted in a complete lack of consistency. In any case, even if GPs or midwives thought that they had presented options to the women, there was plenty of evidence from our interviews that women did not understand that they were being given choices. Most women thought that the system was that they would receive care from the midwifery group practices as a matter of course, even if they thought they had been presented with options by GPs or midwives. In Deptford, the question of choice or options was complicated by the fact that the midwifery group practice was not based in GP surgeries and the women came from a wide variety of GP practices, with differing relationships with midwifery services.

The evidence on how the question of choice of carer was presented to women remains unclear. Many GPs thought that the midwives would be giving women options, and were then surprised to find that they themselves were not seeing pregnant women at all antenatally. When women said that they were offered a choice by midwives, many appeared to feel that the expectation was that they would choose midwifery-led care unless they felt very strongly otherwise or there was a pressing obstetric or medical reason for consultant-led care.

There were clear differences between the areas in the extent to which women chose to have a *home birth,* with nearly 60 per cent of the women we interviewed in Deptford saying they chose a home birth at their first consultation with the midwifery group practice, compared with less than one fifth in Lewisham and only 5 per cent in Ashford. But it would be far too simplistic to assume that women choose home births when they are offered the choice, or that it is the relative lack of availability which limits women's choice.

There were many indications that women sought out the Deptford midwives because of their reputation for encouraging home births. The interviews did not show any great enthusiasm among women for home births in other areas, and, indeed, even in Deptford among those choosing home births, there was evidence that some women felt pressurised, however subtly, into choosing home births because of the enthusiasm of the midwives. On the other hand, there were many indications that women chose hospital births for exactly the same reasons of safety that most GPs and consultant obstetricians favoured hospital births.

We saw how women might opt for a home birth because of poor previous experience of hospital births, showing again how important it is to assess the reasons for opting for what might be a less safe type of care provided in a caring environment by trusted, familiar professionals against a safer care provided in what is perceived to be a poor or hostile environment by unknown and less caring professionals.

Most women in Lewisham and Deptford received most of their *antenatal care* in their own homes, whereas the pattern in Ashford was for most antenatal care to be given by the midwives in the GPs' surgeries in which they were based. The question of choice is interesting here, since the Lewisham and Deptford women felt that they were actually being offered home visits rather than a choice of being visited at home or having the consultation elsewhere. The choice was, in fact, being exercised by the midwife in offering the home visits.

Considerable *choice over timing of consultations* was offered to many women in Lewisham and Deptford, and there were clear indications that the suspicions by GPs that women were receiving evening or weekend visits at home at their convenience were well-founded. It was not surprising that many women valued the flexibility of the midwives in fitting in with their choices, but the question must be asked whether such a system is either sustainable or replicable, not to mention the resource implications. Perhaps even more important is the question of why women who were not ill should receive home visits from midwives when GPs were finding home visits more and more difficult to sustain.

The question of *choices in intrapartum care* centred to a large extent on pain control and circumstances in labour. Modes of delivery, although discussed with women, were often dictated by clinical factors, even though most women were said by midwives to have 'chosen' normal vaginal deliveries. Women in Deptford were much more likely than others to have chosen minimum pain control or water births. Again it is unclear how the options were put to the women and there were indications that women with particular preferences might have sought out the Deptford practice because of the reputation of the midwives.

The question of whether women had been offered the *choice of seeing a consultant obstetrician* at least once in their pregnancy, as recommended in *Changing Childbirth,* was difficult to answer conclusively. Differing evidence came from the women and the midwives.

The women who had seen a consultant obstetrician reported that they had usually done so as a matter of course in that their previous or present medical or obstetric history or condition indicated the need. There were different interpretations among the women interviewed antenatally about whether they had been offered the choice or opportunity of seeing a consultant obstetrician, ranging from nearly 60 per cent of the Ashford women to 40 per cent of the Lewisham women to less than 30 per cent of the Deptford women. However, a higher proportion of the Deptford women than in the other two areas had actually seen a consultant or other hospital doctor in the early antenatal period.

There was difficulty in interpreting the evidence from the midwives about how they presented to women the choice of 'lead professional', the question of whether women were offered the opportunity or choice of seeing a consultant obstetrician, and the extent to which the midwives referred women to consultant obstetricians. It could be argued that the question of whether women are offered the choice of seeing a consultant obstetrician should be inextricably connected to their medical or obstetric needs. Where there is a demonstrated need for consultant care or referral to consultant, the question of women's choice might appear to be secondary.

In Ashford there were clear protocols for assigning women to midwife or consultant care which should have ensured that 'high risk' women would automatically have been under the care of a consultant obstetrician. However, as our analysis shows, a high proportion of Ashford women were offered a choice of lead professional by the midwives and chose midwife-led care, even though they were considered to be 'high risk' cases. We have seen that this led to overload and duplication of effort in the JACANES midwifery group practice.

But there were clearly problems arising in whether the midwives were offering all women the choice or opportunity of seeing a consultant obstetrician during pregnancy. The evidence suggests that relatively few 'low-risk' women were offered this choice, and that women who opted for midwife-led care were doing so without fully understanding that this did not mean that they could not see a consultant, or, for that matter, see their GP if they wished.

It is clear that much caution should be used in interpreting what people understand by offering or being offered choice. Throughout the interviews with respondents from all groups, the notion of choice was explored on a number of issues. Much depended on the perspective of those who thought they were offering choice, those who thought choice was being offered by someone else, and the women who thought they were being offered or not being offered choice. There should be much more informed debate and examination of the extent to which true choices can or should be offered in cases where professional judgement should form an element of the decision. There is often a fine line between seeking to empower users of services while at the same time not jeopardising their safety or health.

Clarification of roles and responsibilities of practitioners and professionals

The SETRHA initiative set out to look at the assumptions that midwifery group practices would reduce duplication of services to women and that there would be clarification of roles and responsibilities of practitioners and professionals.

The evidence suggests that the midwifery group practices, through concentrating the maternity care of women in the hands of one group of professionals, did succeed in reducing the number of consultations with different professionals experienced by women who had had previous pregnancies. It does not, however, necessarily follow that consultations with different professionals always duplicate effort and are therefore undesirable. It clearly depends on a number of factors, including the point of the consultation, the expertise needed and brought to the consultation, and the extent to which the consultations with different professionals are seen as complementary and part of a shared or planned care package.

What appears to have happened through the development of the midwifery group practices is that women were much less likely to see a number of different midwives or other hospital staff in their antenatal care. They found this of positive benefit, and the continuity of care from a named midwife or midwives was much appreciated. However, in addition, women were much less likely to have seen their GPs during the antenatal and postnatal period than had previously been the practice. The women were much less clear about whether this was of benefit to them, but the GPs were generally unhappy about the extent to which their role in maternity care had been eroded, to the point of extinction in some cases.

It could therefore be argued that the desire to eliminate duplication of services had resulted in the replacement of shared and complementary maternity care from professionals with different skills, by care monopolised by one set of professionals. It was certainly the view of most of the GPs interviewed that this could lead not only to less good holistic health care for women during pregnancy and postnatally, but also potentially to less good maternity care, leaving aside the question of the impact on GPs and other professionals and practitioners themselves. There are important issues to be examined here in looking at the relative roles and responsibilities of practitioners and professionals.

There must be considerable doubt about the extent to which the development of the midwifery group practices clarified the roles and responsibilities of practitioners and professionals. Much of the evidence presented in this report points in the other direction. The underlying debate throughout this report of the meaning of 'lead professional' serves to illustrate the potential muddle and lack of accountability which could follow from a lack of clarity about roles and responsibilities. Indeed, far from clarifying roles and responsibilities, the report presents plenty of evidence to suggest that the development of the midwifery group practices created or highlighted tensions between different professionals which were, in some instances, detrimental to the delivery of good services.

Perhaps the most important of these centred on the feeling of exclusion by the GPs, particularly those in the 'host practices'. Many GPs were concerned about the lack of contact between them and their pregnant patients, resulting in lost opportunities to build up good relationships with women which they considered desirable for the future general health care of the family; the loss or deterioration of their own skills in antenatal, intrapartum and postnatal care; and a general sense that the midwifery group practices, far from offering women choice of care and carer, had actually removed choice and had resulted in midwife-only care. Although GPs recognised and acknowledged the skills and expertise of individual midwives, most had strong reservations about the ways in which the schemes had been planned and developed, the lack of clear protocols on roles and responsibilities, the lack of monitoring of protocols, the ways in which the midwifery group practices had been managed, and the impact on their own work and relationships with their patients. In addition, many had concerns about the impact on the midwives themselves, the extent to which the type of services offered by midwives could raise expectations of health care services which could not be delivered by other professionals, for example, home visits, and the possibility that two-tier services would be developed. They were particularly concerned that not all midwives might be of the same high calibre, dedication and commitment as those in the midwifery group practices, and that assumptions might be made about the replicability of the model of care without taking this fully into account. The views of the GPs might be challenged by many midwives.

The danger of the development of a two-tier service was illustrated in other instances of a lack of clarification of roles and responsibilities which appeared to have been associated with the development of the midwifery group practices. There was disquieting evidence from the women of breakdowns in liaison and relationships between hospital staff and the midwifery group practices, with the result that women were regarded as the responsibility of the midwifery group practices and not given the necessary care by other staff. This was reported by a number of women and clearly led to unhappy, and potentially dangerous, situations. These problems were also recognised by the midwifery group practice midwives.

There are other aspects here which should be explored by those who are thinking of extending the role of midwives or developing midwifery group practices. The question of responsibility and accountability, particularly legal accountability, is of increasing importance in obstetrics and maternity care. The evidence from this report, both from women and professionals, of the extent to which the women were regarded as the responsibility of midwives within the midwifery group practices has fundamental implications if something goes wrong. For example, women gave examples of being ignored or neglected in hospital by members of staff, including medical staff. But what would happen if members of hospital staff, including medical staff, failed to give care in an obstetric emergency because the 'lead professional' was not available? On the other hand, what would happen if medical staff failed to intervene in an obstetric emergency because of the presence of the 'lead professional' who was a midwife within the midwifery group practice? There are a number of vitally important issues in terms of accountability which need urgent consideration.

Most consultant obstetricians and GPs interviewed appeared unclear on whether protocols were in place which outlined the respective roles and responsibilities of staff providing care to the women involved in the schemes. There was certainly a lack of clarity about who was ultimately responsible and accountable for women's care.

It is clearly of the utmost importance that respective roles and responsibilities between all medical, midwifery and nursing staff are clarified and that protocols are developed and monitored to ensure that the type of neglect through lack of clarification of roles described by women in this report cannot occur. But there are further urgent needs, including the recognition that protocols need to be constantly reviewed to ensure that they cover all eventualities in new and developing models of practice in maternity care. There were perhaps too many examples in this report not only of a failure to adhere to protocols even where they existed but also of a failure to ensure that proper protocols were in place to cover unexplored territory and developing roles and responsibilities. It should be absolutely clear where the ultimate responsibility for the care and safety of all women and babies lies – in all situations and in all locations.

Self-esteem of midwives

One of the assumptions of SETRHA in setting up the initiative was that the self-esteem of midwives would be improved through working in midwifery group practices, thereby impacting on the quality of care.

There can be no doubt that most of the midwives in all three areas stressed many instances of increased self-esteem and job satisfaction through working in midwifery group practices, particularly in comparison with their previous work experience, whether in hospital or in the community. These related to four main areas: increased job satisfaction in terms of the way they were able to use and demonstrate their skills; increased confidence in their own abilities; being able to get to know and form close relationships with the women to whom they gave care; and working in a supportive network of midwives of similar skills with a shared philosophy.

The increased job satisfaction from using their skills stemmed from the fact that the midwives felt more in control, had more responsibility, greater autonomy, had a known caseload and were able to make fuller use both of their midwifery skills and other skills. They liked being able to give more 'holistic care' to women, instead of carrying out more fragmented midwifery tasks. They liked the continuity of care they could offer, through the whole of the antenatal, intrapartum and postnatal period, which gave them the opportunity to use all their midwifery skills. Midwives who had had little or no experience of home births also felt progressively more confident in their ability to handle these. In general, the midwives welcomed being able to plan their own days and decide how they would allocate their time and visits. This flexibility was of considerable importance to those who were used to more structured ways of working.

Some recognised that greater autonomy brought greater responsibility and the need for continuing clinical vigilance and awareness. At the same time, the increasing responsibility and use of their skills meant that midwives felt more confident in their dealings with other professionals, particularly consultant obstetricians and GPs. On the other hand, it was clear that in all three areas, relationships with some professionals were much better than with others, and that the increased confidence among midwives was not necessarily appreciated or even recognised by some key professionals.

Most midwives felt that the closer relationships they were able to build with women through the continuity of care offered by the midwifery group practices were a source of great job satisfaction. They liked the feeling of 'empowering' women, working in partnership with women and offering them positive birth experiences, although some recognised the dangers of creating dependent relationships which were difficult to sustain, even during the pregnancy and birth, not to mention the problems of letting go after the postnatal period.

It was agreed that working in a midwifery group practice, although regarded as a mainly positive experience by most midwives interviewed, was not without its problems, some of which led to considerable tensions. There were certainly seen to be advantages in working with midwives who shared the same philosophy and were generally seen to have similar levels of skills, which engendered trust and confidence in sharing the care of women. The support offered by the midwives to each other, both in practical and emotional terms was greatly valued.

Even so, there were clear indications in all three practices that choosing and finding group members who were compatible and trusted working partners was not always easy, even among highly motivated midwives such as these. Sharing a philosophy is not enough to ensure harmonious working relationships, as was demonstrated by the fact that one of the midwifery practices called in an outside counsellor to help them resolve their differences.

It was quite clear, however, that although most midwives had achieved greater self-esteem through the midwifery group practices, there had been considerable costs to many of them in personal terms, particularly in relation to their personal lives. Most commented on the extent to which the demands on them through the increased working commitment had impinged on their domestic lives, and there were many warning signals about potential problems with family life through working in this way. It is not unreasonable to expect that many midwives would not wish, or be able, to offer such dedication and time commitment.

Most midwives also pointed to times when they had felt less than completely in control of their practice, simply because of fatigue, and some of the illustrations given both by the midwives themselves and the women we interviewed suggest that safety levels of working time might not always have been closely observed by dedicated practitioners.

Views of women on their experience of the midwifery group practices

This report gives abundant evidence that the majority of women using all three midwifery group practices were satisfied with most aspects of the care and services they received from the midwives, measured on a number of different indicators and covering the full range of services offered by the practices in the antenatal, intrapartum and postnatal periods.

The interviews with the women gave many examples illustrating good practice, particularly in the manner but also in the content of the care which was offered by the midwives. We have quoted from the interviews extensively, since it is only by listening to the voices of those who experience the care, and paying close attention to the words that they themselves use in describing their experience, that the real needs and views of users of services can be established.

An important question which should be asked in an evaluation of this kind is whether there was anything reported by the women in describing good care that was unique to maternity services, or whether the ingredients of good care described should be the goal of all services. In asking this question, however, it must be asked whether care of the type described, with all its emphasis on close personal relationships, enormous flexibility and accessibility, home visiting and so on, is replicable even within maternity services, not to mention more general health services.

It is also important to disentangle the elements of the care given by the midwifery group practices which were particularly appreciated by the women and to assess to what extent these were related more to the manner than to the content of the care. It has long been recognised that excellent technical care can be given by those with no interpersonal skills at all, while charming professionals can be technically and professionally far less competent and yet be judged by users to have delivered a good service.

There can be no doubt that many of the reasons given by the women for regarding the midwifery group practices as good services centred on the manner in which they were treated by the midwives. The interviews covered a wide range of topics, but throughout the answers it was clear that women liked being treated with respect, like adults, as individuals; they liked being given confidence in themselves, a feeling of being in control, of independence; they liked feeling that they could trust their midwives, that their midwife would be their advocate, that their midwife was their 'friend' and was 'on their side'. They liked the flexibility and accessibility of the midwives, the quick response and ease of contact, and the amount of time that the midwives gave them. The relationships described were often very close. The woman who said that 'every woman falls in love with her midwife' might have been at one end of the spectrum but certainly captured an element of the type of relationships with midwives described by many of the women interviewed for this study.

But how good was the actual care? And could the women judge the expertise and clinical practice of the midwives? Could they judge whether the advice being given by the midwives was correct? Could they really exercise informed choice on important clinical issues? Did they actually have enough information? Did the midwives always give them all the information they needed? It is almost impossible to know. There were certainly indications that some women were surprised by the fact that they did not have a home birth as planned, or that the pain control they selected proved inadequate, or that their labour was much quicker or more complicated than they expected. But this does not necessarily mean that they were not informed of all possibilities. And it does not mean that the care and expertise offered by the midwives was in any way different from the care and expertise offered by other professionals.

Essentially, the interviews with the women showed a high degree of appreciation of the personal qualities and type of care provided by the midwifery group practices. But, as we have noted time and again in the report, in many cases the comparison was with previous experience and the high level of satisfaction was more an indictment of the manner and organisation of the care offered in hospitals in particular than a blanket endorsement of midwifery group practices as a model of care. We should also underline the fact that women who had received previous care from individual midwives who were now members of the midwifery group practices observed no discernible differences in the type or manner of care they had been offered in their current pregnancies from that which they had received before from the same midwife. It has always been recognised that much depends on the personalities and skills of individual professionals. Care should be taken in extrapolating from the evidence of high levels of consumer satisfaction with groups of dedicated and committed midwives who chose to come together to provide a particular model of care. The model in itself may not be the main ingredient of success.

Resource issues

The question of resources has run throughout this report and links very closely with the last section. One of the main criteria in judging the success of the schemes must be whether they delivered good quality care at a cost acceptable to the purchasing authorities. It is important to remember the comment of the consultant obstetrician who observed, 'It's not successful if they're nice but you can't afford them...'

We were asked to examine issues of costs and effectiveness, but, as we show in detail in Chapters 2 and 9, our approach had to be restricted to providing cost descriptions and to make most of our comparisons on the basis of resources and not costs. The data on costs were simply not robust enough to conduct proper cost-effectiveness exercises, and detailed comparisons between the costs of the three midwifery group practices were inappropriate because the cost bases were quite different. There were a variety of reasons for this, some of which were related to the overall extent to which the internal market in health care had developed in each of the districts, and others of which were related more closely to the differences and intricacies of costing and measuring midwifery and maternity services both in general and in the particular districts.

They included key problems in data availability and quality; uncertainty among respondents about cost issues; discrepancies in different versions of events and/or figures among purchasers and providers; different ways of defining or purchasing episodes of care; different ways of calculating unit costs, particularly in the apportioning of overheads, cross-subsidisation and hidden overheads; and different interpretations of whether price covered costs.

In addition, an underlying theme throughout this study was the extent to which there was potential or actual duplication of costs when women received care from a number of different agencies. This was of particular importance when women had hospital treatment and/or births but most of their antenatal or postnatal maternity care was provided under a different contract, and, of course, when women transferred from one midwifery practice to another. None of this takes into account the costs of GP obstetric care.

All these issues must be taken into account by those who are planning the development of maternity services. In our evaluation we were struck time and again by the paucity of reliable cost data available to those who were drawing up contracts. We also noted difficulties in extracting reliable data which demonstrated the real resource implications of the use of the midwives' time. We give details in the report of different rota/on-call arrangements; different ways in which on-call was reimbursed; and different ways of accounting for time used. We note the extent to which home visiting was common in Deptford and Lewisham but not in Ashford. We note the wide variations in travel costs.

There can be no doubt that it was difficult to make a comprehensive assessment of the true resource implications of the midwifery group practices in Lewisham and Ashford, if only because the midwives did not always regard their out-of-hours work with their own women as 'duty'. In addition, the overload on the Ashford midwives for the first nine or ten months of the monitoring period was such that it was impossible to disentangle what kind of caseload was feasible.

The true costs and resource implications of the Deptford midwifery group practice were even more difficult to assess. We have already noted in this chapter that they were having to act as a small business as well as a midwifery group practice, with all the resource implications of using the time and energy of their professional staff in establishing business, building up customers, negotiating contracts, establishing a team and so on, rather than focusing on delivering a service of sufficient capacity to satisfy the requirements in terms of numbers laid down by SETRHA when it set up the pilot projects. Indeed the Deptford midwifery group practice never reached the required numbers during the monitoring period, nor did it satisfy all the requirements of its commissioners in reaching its target population.

We concluded that, for the many reasons stated, it was not possible to provide a clear-cut and comprehensive assessment of the costs of the midwifery group practice models as established in all three pilot sites. We can say, however, that in terms of resources they provided more midwife-intensive practice than traditional midwifery practice in both the community and in hospitals, and, on this basis, were more expensive both in cost terms and in real resource terms. This has implications for rolling out the models more widely, and, in planning for this transition, both the midwifery managers in Lewisham and Ashford envisaged an increase in the staffing levels and budget required.

So far as any cost-effectiveness assessment of the pilot midwifery group practice projects is concerned we concluded that this must necessarily be based on relatively 'soft' data in the absence of robust information on the true costs. Consideration should be given to whether the undoubtedly increased resource implications were offset by gains to women in terms of satisfaction with the service they were given and by gains to the midwives in increasing their job-satisfaction, albeit at personal costs in terms of fatigue and overload. Other cost and resource implications and other benefits and disbenefits have been discussed in the report and in this chapter. They should all be taken into account by those who have responsibility for planning services and for 'rolling out' *Changing Childbirth*. It should be apparent that a simple cost-benefit formula does not exist.

Evaluating and monitoring innovatory practice

There are fundamental questions to be answered about how best to ensure proper monitoring and evaluation of midwifery services in general, and services of an innovatory type in particular. There is a clear need to ensure not only that effective monitoring systems are in place before services are implemented but also that management systems are in place to ensure that changes are made as soon as problems start to arise. This may sound an obvious statement, but our experience as independent evaluators has shown us that it does not automatically occur, particularly when service providers are keen to demonstrate that an innovative model is successful.

It was only through the rigorous monitoring agreed with the research team at Policy Studies Institute that the major overload on the midwives in Ashford was demonstrated and then acted upon. Similarly, it was our continuing analysis that provided information to managers of the high numbers in Lewisham and the low numbers in Deptford. It is a cause for concern that it was only through the monitoring of an independent evaluator that attention was drawn to fundamental organisational problems relating to numbers which should have been noted as they were happening.

As the research team commissioned to evaluate these projects, Policy Studies Institute researchers were always concerned to maintain the role of independent evaluators. We often found ourselves at the centre of debates about professional boundaries, territories and roles and responsibilities. We observed claims about practice and outcomes which were not always based on sound or robust evidence. We sometimes found ourselves having to correct information assembled by the midwifery group practices which did not concur with the routine monitoring information they had collected and given to us.

We consider it important that independent assessments are made of innovatory schemes wherever possible, but we recognise that this will often be too expensive or not feasible. However, we would reiterate the points made above that monitoring systems and internal evaluation should always be instituted and controlled by staff other than the service providers themselves. Professionals should provide the services for which they have the expertise and training – in all fields.

Overall assessment

We have concentrated in this discussion of findings on the lessons which can be learnt from the setting up of three midwifery group practice pilot projects by SETRHA. We have examined the assumptions on which the pilot projects were funded and have evaluated as far as possible the outcomes we were asked to investigate. We have concluded that the exercise demonstrated that, in spite of undoubted benefits to women and to midwives, there were many questions raised by the exercise which had not hitherto been properly examined and assessed. These have been explored in detail in this report and in this chapter. They suggest that considerable caution should be exercised before it is assumed that models of this kind are replicable.

This report offers considerable insights into the ingredients of good and caring midwifery practice, but it also gives many warnings about how a failure to recognise or acknowledge the personal and inter-professional costs of organising maternity services in this way may cause more problems than they solve. The report also gives abundant evidence that some of the assumptions about women's choices and women's well-being may not always be rooted in the reality of what women themselves actually want. In their important achievements in moving the delivery of maternity services away from the domination of the 'medical model' and the medical establishment, enthusiasts for midwifery services would be unwise to lose sight of the fact that a good partnership should be maintained between midwives and the medical profession. Recognition among professional groups of the professional skills and expertise of others is an essential part of providing good holistic health care to all users of services.

Appendix A

Midwifery group practices: duty rota and diary exercise tables

Table A.1 Longest number of day shift hours and residual on-call hours for each Lewisham MGP midwife between days off (taken from the MGP duty rota)

	MW 1	MW 2	MW 3	MW 4	MW 5	MW 6	MW 7
Day shift	37½	60	60	52½	67½	75	60
Residual on-call	32	64	48	32	64	80	64
Total: day shift and residual on-call hours	*(69½)*	*(124)*	*(108)*	*(84½)*	*(131½)*	*(155)*	*(124)*

Length of day shift is 7½ hours – from 9am to 5pm (excluding breaks).
Residual on-call is 16 hours (24 hours minus regular day shift time from 9am to 5pm).

Table A.2 Hours spent on diary sheet activities by each Lewisham MGP midwife during the 2-week diary exercise period

	Direct care	Phone	Meetings	Travel	Admin	Misc	Recorded time	Scheduled time
MW 1	37¾	4¼	11½	7	9	3¾	73¼	75
MW 2	66	2	1	6	11	½	86½	60
MW 3	58½	3¾	5	4½	9	1¼	82	60
MW 4	72	1¼	4¼	22½	4½	2	106½	75
MW 5	50½	8½	4¾	13¼	21¾	13¾	112½	75
MW 6	31¼	7¾	8½	11	18¾	16¾	94	82½
MW 7	46	8½	8½	20½	14½	1½	99½	75
Mean	*51¾*	*5¼*	*6¼*	*12*	*12¾*	*5¾*	*93*	*71¾*
Total hours:	*(362)*	*(36)*	*(43½)*	*(84¾)*	*(88½)*	*(39½)*	*(654¼)*	*(502½)*

Recorded time corresponds to the amount of time attributed to activities on the diary sheets.
Scheduled time is the time that midwives were scheduled to work (regular day shift only) taken from the duty rota during the 2-week diary exercise period.

Table A.3   Hours spent on direct care activities by each Lewisham MGP
midwife during the 2-week diary exercise period

	Booking	Ante natal	Intra partum	Post natal	Special appts	Classes	Total
MW 1	0	17	13	7¾	0	0	37¾
MW 2	1	8¼	39½	14¾	2½	0	66
MW 3	4	10	25½	14½	0	4½	58½
MW 4	7	15¼	19¾	26	2	2	72
MW 5	3¼	8	26½	10	1¼	1½	50½
MW 6	5½	11¾	5½	8	½	0	31¼
MW 7	1½	18	6	20½	0	0	46
Mean	3¼	12½	19½	14½	*	1¼	51¾
Total hours:	*(22¼)*	*(88¼)*	*(135¾)*	*(101½)*	*(6¼)*	*(8)*	*(362)*

* equals less than 1 hour

Table A.4   Longest number of day shift hours and residual on-call hours for
each Ashford MGP midwife between days off (taken from the
MGP duty rota)

	MW 1	MW 2	MW 3	MW 4	MW 5	MW 6	MW 7
Day shift	32	24	48	24	48	40	32
Residual on-call	20½	24½	30	15	30	24½	24½
Total: day shift and residual on-call hours	*(52½)*	*(48½)*	*(78)*	*(39)*	*(78)*	*(64½)*	*(56½)*

Length of day shift is 8 hours from 8am to 5pm (excluding breaks).
Residual on-call is 5½ hours for 'on-call 1' and 9½ hours for 'on-call 2'.

Table A.5 Hours spent on diary sheet activities by each Ashford MGP midwife during the 2-week diary exercise period

	Direct care	Phone	Meetings	Travel	Admin	Misc	Recorded time	Scheduled time
MW 1	31½	8¾	6½	11½	13½	30¼	102	48
MW 2	44¼	5½	4	7¾	6¼	0	67¾	40
MW 3	26¼	2	9	5	13½	¼	56	56
MW 4	13½	2½	15	8	7½	5	51½	32
MW 5	46	5½	10¾	7¾	7½	2½	80	80
MW 6	35½	4½	3½	4¾	12	5	65¼	64
MW 7	29	3	8¼	11	14½	11½	77¼	64
Mean	32¼	4½	8¼	8	10¾	7¾	71½	54¾
Total hours:	*(226)*	*(31¾)*	*(57)*	*(55¾)*	*(74¾)*	*(54½)*	*(499¾)*	*(384)*

Recorded time corresponds to the amount of time attributed to activities on the diary sheets.
Scheduled time is the time that midwives were scheduled to work (regular day shift only) taken from the duty rota during the 2-week diary exercise period.

Table A.6 Hours spent on direct care activities by each Ashford MGP midwife during the 2-week diary exercise period

	Booking	Ante natal	Intra partum	Post natal	Special appts	Classes	Total
MW 1	6	16	4¼	3	¼	2	31½
MW 2	2	6	20½	8¼	1½	6	44¼
MW 3	3¾	14	0	8½	0	0	26¼
MW 4	0	1	4½	6¾	0	1¼	13½
MW 5	5	8¼	19½	10¾	0	2½	46
MW 6	0	13¾	7	10¾	0	4	35½
MW 7	4	13	0	9	0	3	29
Mean	*3*	*10¼*	*8*	*8¼*	*	*2¾*	*32¼*
Total hours:	*(20¾)*	*(72)*	*(55¾)*	*(57)*	*(1¾)*	*(18¾)*	*(226)*

Table A.7 Hours spent on diary sheet activities by each Deptford MGP midwife during the 2-week diary exercise period

	Direct care	Phone	Meetings	Travel	Admin	Misc	Breaks	Total
MW 1	64½	12½	16¾	17	7	8	0	125¾
MW 3	62¼	12	10½	15	6	4	0	109¾
MW 4	42	12¼	11½	16½	13¾	7	3½	106½
MW 5	31¾	6	6½	6	4¼	½	¾	55¾
MW 9	51¾	9¼	7¼	11½	¼	2	0	82
Mean	*50½*	*10½*	*10½*	*13¼*	*6¼*	*4¼*	*	*96*
Total hours:	*(252¼)*	*(52)*	*(52½)*	*(66)*	*(31¼)*	*(21½)*	*(4¼)*	*(479¾)*
ORH	*80¾*	*19¾*	*6*	*15½*	*9¾*	*0*	*0*	*131¾*

Outside regular hours (ORH) is from 5pm to 9am.
Midwives 02, 06, 07 and 08 left the MGP before this exercise was carried out.

Table A.8 Hours spent on direct care activities by each Deptford MGP midwife during the 2-week diary exercise period

	Booking	Ante natal	Intra partum	Post natal	Special appts	Classes	Total
MW 1	2½	24¾	10½	16¼	8	2½	64½
MW 3	8½	14¾	22¼	12¼	1	3½	62¼
MW 4	4¼	3¾	10¾	18½	0	4¾	42
MW 5	5¼	11	4½	3	2	6	31¾
MW 9	0	14¼	24	11½	0	2	51¾
Mean	4	13¾	14½	12¼	2¼	3¾	50½
Total hours:	*(20½)*	*(68½)*	*(72)*	*(61½)*	*(11)*	*(18¾)*	*(252¼)*
ORH	*5¾*	*12*	*34¾*	*8*	*8*	*12¼*	*80¾*

Outside regular hours (ORH) is from 5pm to 9am.
Midwives 02, 06, 07 and 08 left the MGP before this exercise was carried out.

Appendix B

JACANES on-call cover arrangements

Continuous cover for women was provided through a combination of regular day shift and three on-call cover arrangements.

'*On-call 1*' – provided by 1 midwife from 7.30 am until 10 pm. During this time the midwife cared for clients on her own caseload and provided on-call cover for midwives who were off-duty or otherwise unavailable.

'*On-call 2*' – provided by 1 midwife and was always preceded by a regular day shift from 8 am until 5 pm. Following a break from 5 pm until 10 pm the on-call 2 midwife provided cover from 10 pm until 7.30 am.

The *third on-call* cover arrangement involved providing on-call cover outside regular day shift hours for women on the midwife's caseload. Midwives could provide on-call cover for their own clients for up to 2 nights each fortnight. However, this on-call arrangement was relatively flexible and was based on the idea that if a midwife had been particularly busy, she could opt out of providing cover to women on her own caseload by handing over to the midwife providing general on-call cover.

Midwives did not provide on-call cover for their own clients on or before a day-off or if assigned a night off on the duty rota. A more limited form of on-call cover was introduced following a regular day shift for midwives scheduled on an 'on-call 1' the next day. In such instances the midwife continued to provide on-call cover for women on her own caseload after the end of the regular day shift at 5 pm until 10 pm. The midwife then switched off her mobile phone to ensure that she was not called upon during the night.

Appendix C

Characteristics of service users and outcome details for women who booked with MGP midwives before April 1994

In Chapter 3 we gave details of the monitoring exercise carried out for all women who received MGP care from 1 April 1994 to 30 September 1995. We noted that the MGPs did not start from scratch and that each brought a number of women with them who had booked with the MGP midwives before 1 April 1994. The aim of this appendix is to present a profile of this group of service users and their main characteristics. The outcome of pregnancy for this group of women is also given. Table 3.1 gives details of the monitoring data collected for all women who received MGP care, including those who booked with the MGPs both before and after April 1994 and Table 3.5 shows the monthly deliveries for each MGP for both groups of women.

Our monitoring exercise started on 1 April 1994, so that first consultation forms for women who had booked with MGP midwives *before* 1 April 1994 were completed at a point in pregnancy when many of them had already received a substantial amount of antenatal care. However, this information enables us to highlight similarities and differences between women who booked with the MGP midwives before and after 1 April 1994. The following discussion should be looked at in conjunction with the information presented in Chapter 3 on the characteristics of the women who booked with the MGPs during the monitoring period.

One of the main messages from the data is that the two groups of women booking before and after April 1994 in both Lewisham and in Ashford were similar in many respects, showing that both these MGPs provided a service to similar groups of women irrespective of when they booked. In contrast, women booking with the Deptford MGP before and after April 1994 showed some differences in relation to characteristics such as ethnic group, social class and housing status. However, despite these differences the two groups of women booking with the Deptford

MGP were more similar to each other than to women booking with the other MGPs.

Age profile of service users

Table C.1 shows the age profile of service users in each of the three areas and indicates that women who booked with the MGP midwives before April 1994 were similar in age profile to the women who booked after April 1994. The average age of women booking with the MGP midwives before April 1994 was higher in Deptford (31.1 years) than in Ashford (27.3 years) and Lewisham (28.9 years). This reflected the pattern found among the women who booked with the respective MGPs after April 1994.

Table C.1   Age of women who booked with the MGPs before April 1994

			column percentages
	Lewisham	Ashford	Deptford
16-19	5	6	3
20-24	18	24	7
25-29	24	37	20
30-34	37	24	46
35-39	14	7	19
40 plus	1	1	4
n.a.	1	*	1
Mean age	28.9	27.3	31.3
Base: Pre-April 1994 bookings (146)		*(234)*	*(70)*

* equals less than 1 per cent

Women who booked with MGP midwives before April 1994 in Ashford were twice as likely to be under 30 as women in Deptford. 30 per cent of the women in Ashford were under 25 compared with 23 per cent of women in Lewisham and only 10 per cent in Deptford. 20 per cent of women in Deptford were 25–29 years compared with around a quarter of the women in Lewisham (24 per cent) and over a third of the women in Ashford (37 per cent).

As we found among the women booking in the monitoring period, the Deptford MGP attracted a high proportion of women who were 30 years and over. Women in Deptford were over twice as likely to be 30 years or over (69 per cent) as women in Ashford (32 per cent). 52 per cent of the Lewisham women were 30 or over.

Marital status

A similar pattern in relation to marital status was found for women who booked with the midwives before and after April 1994. Women who had booked with the MGP midwives before April 1994 in Deptford were more likely to be living as married (33 per cent) than women who booked after April 1994 (27 per cent), but otherwise there was little difference between women booking before and during the monitoring period in the other two areas (Table C.2). 21 per cent of the women who booked with a Lewisham MGP midwife before April 1994 were living as married compared with 24 per cent of women in Ashford.

Table C.2   Marital status of women who booked with the MGPs before April 1994

column percentages

	Lewisham	Ashford	Deptford
Single	22	5	13
Married	56	69	53
Living as married	21	24	33
Widowed	0	0	0
Divorced	0	1	0
Separated	1	1	0
n.a.	0	*	1
Base: Pre-April 1994 bookings (146)		*(234)*	*(70)*

The pre-April 1994 group of women in Ashford were more likely to be married and less likely to be single than women elsewhere. Over two-thirds of the women in Ashford (69 per cent) were married, compared with over half the women in Lewisham (56 per cent) and Deptford (53 per cent). 22 per cent of the women in Lewisham were single compared with only 5 per cent in Ashford. A lower proportion of women booking before April 1994 were single (13 per cent) in Deptford compared with women booking with the Deptford MGP during the monitoring period (21 per cent).

Social class and occupation

a) *Women's occupation*

Table C.3 shows that women in Deptford who booked before April 1994 were three times more likely to be in professional and managerial occupations (60 per cent) than women in Ashford (18 per cent) and Lewisham

(19 per cent). This table shows the extent to which midwives in the Deptford MGP had attracted women from non-manual occupations before the pilot projects were set up. This could be partly explained by the fact that the MGP had provided a service mainly to self-financing clients before NHS contracts were negotiated. However, even with the contractual eligibility criteria imposed for the MGP service, women booking with the Deptford MGP after April 1994 were also much more likely to be in non-manual occupations than women elsewhere.

Table C.3　Social class/occupation of women who booked with MGPs and their partners before April 1994

column percentages

	Women			Partners		
	Lew	Ash	Dept	Lew	Ash	Dept
Professional I	5	2	6	6	6	24
Intermediate II	14	16	54	22	21	34
Skilled non-manual III N	35	24	7	13	8	10
Skilled manual III M	2	2	4	27	27	4
Semi-skilled IV	4	4	1	10	10	3
Unskilled V	1	3	0	3	10	0
Student	2	2	6	2	2	6
Armed Forces	0	0	0	1	1	0
Keeping house/Mother	26	41	11	0	*	0
Unemployed	10	3	9	12	11	10
n.a.	1	2	1	3	3	9
Base: Pre-April 1994 *bookings*	*(146)*	*(234)*	*(70)*	*(146)*	*(234)*	*(70)*

A small proportion of women in all areas were in skilled manual, semi-skilled and unskilled occupations. Women in skilled non-manual occupations featured more in Lewisham (35 per cent) and Ashford (24 per cent) than in Deptford (7 per cent).

Women in Ashford were nearly four times more likely to be housewives or mothers than women in Deptford (11 per cent). Over a quarter of women in Lewisham (26 per cent) reported this. A similar pattern was found among women who booked after April 1994. There were rather more students in Deptford than elsewhere. Around the same proportion of women were reported to be unemployed in Deptford (9 per cent) and Lewisham (10 per cent) compared with Ashford (3 per cent).

b) Partner's occupation

Table C.3 shows that almost the same proportion of partners were in professional and managerial occupations in Lewisham (28 per cent) and Ashford (27 per cent): a similar proportion to that found during the monitoring period. However, 58 per cent of women who booked with the Deptford MGP before the monitoring period had partners in professional and managerial occupations compared with 49 per cent during the monitoring period.

Partners in Lewisham were more likely be in skilled non-manual occupations (13 per cent) than partners in Ashford (8 per cent) and Deptford (10 per cent).

Nearly half the partners in Ashford (47 per cent) were in manual occupations compared with 40 per cent in Lewisham and only 7 per cent in Deptford. The most common occupational category for partners in Lewisham and Ashford (27 per cent) were skilled manual occupations, while in Deptford more partners were in managerial occupations. This finding also mirrors that for partners of women booking during the monitoring period.

Among both groups of partners a similar proportion were unemployed across all areas: 12 per cent in Lewisham, 11 per cent in Ashford and 10 per cent in Deptford.

Ethnic group

Table C.4 shows that the majority of women booking with the MGP midwives before April 1994 were of white ethnic origin. This was much more evident for the women booking with Deptford midwives before April 1994 than for women who booked with the MGP within the monitoring period. Approximately the same proportion of women booking with Ashford and Lewisham MGPs before and during the monitoring period were of white ethnic origin. In contrast, 93 per cent of women booking in Deptford before April 1994 were of white ethnic origin, compared with 73 per cent booking during the monitoring period. This difference may be attributed to the fact that targeting women from ethnic minority groups was set out by local commissioning agencies as part of the eligibility criteria for the MGP service in Deptford.

There was little ethnic diversity among women booking pre-April 1994 in either Ashford or Deptford. 6 per cent of women in Deptford and less than 2 per cent in Ashford were from Black minority groups. 1 per cent of women in Deptford were Vietnamese and 1 per cent were Indian in Ashford.

In Lewisham, women booking with midwives before and during the monitoring period showed a similar ethnic pattern. 24 per cent of women booking pre-April were from non-white ethnic minority groups with 19 per cent of women of the total from Black ethnic minority groups. 23 per cent of women booking after April 1994 were from non-white ethnic minority groups with 18 per cent of women from Black ethnic minority groups alone.

Table C.4   Ethnic group of women who booked with the MGPs before April 1994

column percentages

	Lewisham	Ashford	Deptford
White	76	95	93
Black Caribbean	12	1	3
Black African	6	*	0
Black British	1	0	3
Indian	1	1	0
Pakistani	0	0	0
Bangladeshi	0	0	0
Chinese	1	*	0
Vietnamese	1	0	1
Mixed race	2	0	0
Other	1	1	0
Base: Pre-April 1994 bookings (146)	(234)	(70)

Housing status

The living arrangements of women booking with midwives in Lewisham and Ashford before and during the monitoring period were very similar, but in Deptford pre-April 1994 figures showed a higher proportion of owner-occupiers and private tenants as Table C.5 shows.

Comparing the pre and post-April 1994 bookings, a slightly higher proportion of women booking with MGP midwives before April 1994 in Lewisham (51 per cent) and Ashford (59 per cent) were owner-occupiers, while in Deptford, nearly two-thirds of women were owner-occupiers (64 per cent) compared with over half of the women who booked with the MGP after April 1994. Around the same proportion of women in Lewisham (8 per cent) and Ashford (10 per cent) were private tenants compared with 16 per cent in Deptford. Over a quarter of women in Lewisham (26 per cent) and a fifth in Ashford were council tenants compared with 16 per cent of women in Deptford.

More women in Lewisham were living with relatives than elsewhere which was also found to be the case for women booking within the monitoring period. 9 per cent of women in Lewisham were living with relatives compared with 6 per cent in Ashford and 3 per cent in Deptford. A few women in all areas were reported to have other living arrangements.

Table C.5   Housing status of women who booked with the MGPs before April 1994

column percentages

	Lewisham	Ashford	Deptford
Owner-occupier	51	59	64
Private tenant	8	10	16
Council tenant	26	20	16
Hotel or hostel	1	0	0
Living with relatives	9	6	3
Housing Association	2	1	0
Temporary address	0	*	0
Other living arrangements	1	3	0
n.a.	2	*	0
Base: Pre-April 1994 bookings (146)		*(234)*	*(70)*

Number of previous pregnancies

Table C.6 reinforces the similarities between the women booking in Lewisham and Ashford before and after April 1994 and underlines some of the differences between the women booking with the Deptford midwives before and during the monitoring period. Comparing the two groups, almost the same proportion of women in Ashford (30 per cent) and Lewisham (28 per cent) reported being pregnant for the first time before and during the monitoring period, while 33 per cent of Deptford women booking pre-April 1994 were having first pregnancies compared with 20 per cent of women who booked during the monitoring period.

Table C.6   Previous pregnancies of women who booked with the MGPs before April 1994

column percentages

	Lewisham	Ashford	Deptford
None	28	30	33
1	32	38	30
2	16	17	21
3 plus	23	15	16
Base: Pre-April 1994 bookings (146)		*(234)*	*(70)*

Lead professional

Women booking with the MGP midwives before April 1994 would not have had the same opportunity to choose who they wanted to care for them in pregnancy and for the birth of their babies. However, we were interested in the extent to which there were differences between women who booked with the same MGP at different time periods and between the MGPs themselves.

96 per cent of women in the pre-April 1994 group in Deptford were reported to have had a midwife as lead professional which was similar to women who booked during the monitoring period. However, in Lewisham, 82 per cent of women who booked before April 1994 had a midwife as lead professional compared with 91 per cent of women who had booked after April 1994. The proportion of women booking before April 1994 with a midwife as lead professional seems high and may be attributable to the fact that midwife-led care had already been introduced before the MGP was set up in Lewisham.

In Ashford the picture was almost the reverse for women booking before and after April 1994. For instance, 72 per cent of women booking with an MGP midwife before April 1994 had a consultant obstetrician as lead professional compared with 20 per cent booking after April. 22 per cent of the pre-April group of women had a midwife as lead professional compared with 71 per cent who booked after April 1994.

The figures quoted for post-April 1994 bookings relate to women in all areas who were offered a choice of lead professional.

Planned place of birth

Although women who booked before the monitoring period were less likely to have been offered a choice of place of birth we were still interested in where women had planned to give birth. In fact, they were not very different from women booking after April 1994 who had been offered a choice of place of birth. For instance, 10 per cent of pre-April 1994 women booking in Lewisham had planned to have a home birth compared with 4 per cent in Ashford and 70 per cent in Deptford. 89 per cent of women had planned to have a hospital birth in Ashford, and another 4 per cent planned to deliver in the GP maternity unit in the hospital. 91 per cent of women in Lewisham planned to have a hospital birth but only 23 per cent of women in Deptford. 7 per cent of women in Deptford were reported to be undecided about place of birth at that point.

Location of the first consultation

Given that many of the women had already had their first booking consultation some months before, we asked midwives to complete a first consultation form at the first consultation after 1 April 1994, so that we had full details of all women receiving MGP care during the monitoring period. We envisaged that the form would be completed during a routine antenatal consultation and would not necessarily reflect what happened at a first consultation or booking visit because some of the topics would already have been covered by the midwife.

60 per cent of these consultations were carried out at home in Lewisham, 29 per cent at the GP practice and 9 per cent at the hospital antenatal clinic. 93 per cent of the first consultations were held at the woman's home in Deptford, 5 per cent at the MGP office, 1 per cent at the hospital clinic and 1 per cent at a midwife's home. In contrast, only 23 per cent of first consultations were held at home in Ashford and the remaining 77 per cent were held at the GP practice. This pattern was similar to that found among booking visits in the post-April group of women and underlines the differences in practice adopted by the MGPs in the monitoring period in general.

Time spent on first consultations

Midwives were asked to indicate the length of the first consultations carried out with this group of women after 1 April 1994. We expected that the time spent would be similar to the amount of time spent on second and subsequent consultations among the post-April group of women. However, the data showed that midwives in Deptford spent three times longer (104.2 minutes) on these consultations than midwives in Ashford (26.2 minutes), while midwives in Lewisham spent on average 47 minutes.

If we compare this with the time spent on booking consultations for the post-April 1994 group of women, the Deptford midwives spent a similar amount of time (114.2 minutes), while Lewisham midwives spent an average of 78.1 minutes on first consultations and Ashford midwives spent an average of 55.7 minutes.

As expected, there were marked differences in the average amount of time spent by midwives on this first consultation during the monitoring period with the pre-April 1994 group according to the location of the consultation. For instance, midwives in Lewisham spent nearly three-quarters as much time on first consultations at home (55.7 minutes) than on GP practice-based consultations (32.6 minutes). While the difference was not as marked in Ashford midwives still spent nearly 50 per cent more time on consultations at home (34.7 minutes) than GP practice-based consultations (23.6 minutes). None of the Deptford consultations were carried out at the GP surgery, but Deptford midwives spent twice as long on consultations at the woman's home (108.2 minutes) than on consultations at the MGP office (52 minutes).

Outcome of pregnancy

Midwives were asked to record the outcome of each pregnancy and Table C.7 shows the proportion of outcomes under different category headings. Outcome details were completed by the midwives for 96 per cent of the women in Lewisham, 98 per cent in Ashford and 89 per cent in Deptford, who, according to the records, had booked with the MGP midwives before 1 April 1994.

Table C.7   Outcome of pregnancy of women who booked with the MGPs before April 1994

column percentages

	Lewisham	Ashford	Deptford
Baby alive at discharge from midwife	99	98	98
Born alive but died before discharge	1	*	0
Stillbirth	1	*	2
Miscarriage	0	*	0
Client moved	0	*	0
Base: all pre-April 1994 women with outcome details	*(140)*	*(225)*	*(62)*

Table C.7 shows that all the outcomes completed in Lewisham and Deptford, and all but 2 in Ashford (a miscarriage and a notification of a client moving out of the area) related to maternities.

Appendix D

Accessible care: location and duration of first and subsequent antenatal consultations

The issue of accessible or community-based antenatal care has important implications for the planning, organisation and provision of maternity care. In Chapter 3 of this report we saw that most of the first and subsequent antenatal consultations took place at home in Lewisham and Deptford and at the GP practice in Ashford. This Appendix looks in more detail at the time spent by midwives on antenatal consultations and their location. It is evident from the monitoring information presented in Tables D.1 and D.2 that the MGPs developed different practices in relation to antenatal care, and that midwives from within the same MGPs did not appear to work in the same way. The implications of different approaches within and between the MGPs are noted and discussed in the context of sustainable practice and replicability of the MGP models of care in the concluding chapter.

Duration of first consultations across different locations

Chapter 3 showed that most of the first consultations carried out in Lewisham (81 per cent) and Deptford (88 per cent) took place at home while in Ashford most took place at local GP practices (81 per cent). Table D.1 shows that the Deptford MGP spent the most time and the Ashford MGP spent the least time on consultations in all locations.

The *Lewisham* MGP spent, on average, 40 per cent more time on home-based consultations than on GP practice-based consultations. This has clear resource implications if most of the consultations take place at home, which they did.

The difference in time spent by the *Ashford* MGP on home-based and GP practice-based consultations was less marked: 15 per cent more time was spent on home-based consultations than on GP practice-based consultations. But given that the Ashford MGP spent consistently less time on first consultations than other MGPs, this minimises any differences attributed to location.

The *Deptford* MGP spent the most time on home and hospital-based first consultations. Given that the majority of first consultations took place at home it is clear that this investment of time might only be sustainable if the MGP continued to operate at less than full capacity. Again there are resource implications in such a high level of time input in home-based consultations.

Table D.1   Average length of time spent by MGPs on first consultations in different locations

mean time in minutes

	Lewisham	Ashford	Deptford
Location			
Home	81.7	62.1	116.0
(Number of consultations)	(407)	(97)	(153)
Hospital	72.4	70.0	117.5
(Number of consultations)	(19)	(3)	(2)
GP practice	58.1	54.2	90.0
(Number of consultations)	(61)	(450)	(1)
Albany Centre	0	0	93.3
(Number of consultations)	(0)	(0)	(9)
n.a.	(11)	(5)	(3)
All locations of first consultations	*78.1*	*55.7*	*114*
(Number of consultations)	*(498)*	*(555)*	*(168)*

Time spent by individual midwives on first consultations

We saw in Chapter 3 that the Deptford MGP spent, on average, twice as long (114 minutes) on first consultations than midwives in Ashford (55.7 minutes) and 50 per cent more time than midwives in Lewisham (78.1 minutes). We looked at the time spent on consultations by individual midwives to see if there were any differences within the MGPs.

The monitoring information revealed that midwives from the same MGPs operated quite differently in relation to the time they spent on consultations. In addition, the time differences could not be fully explained by the overall number of first consultations that the midwives carried out.

Lewisham: the average amount of time spent by individual midwives on first consultations ranged from 61 to 96 minutes. The midwife who spent the longest time on first consultations did so consistently, spending over an hour on 87 per cent of all the first consultations she carried out. In contrast, the midwife who recorded the least time spent over an hour on only 29 per cent of her first consultations.

Ashford: over half the midwives spent a similar amount of time on first consultations while the remainder spent either much more or much less time. The average time spent on first consultations ranged from 43.2 to 74.7 minutes. The midwife who spent the longest time spent over one hour on 55 per cent of all her first consultations compared with the midwife recording the least time who spent over one hour on only 5 per cent of her first consultations.

Deptford: the time spent by individual midwives on first consultations ranged from 97.1 to 120.5 minutes. Over 95 per cent of the first consultations carried out by the Deptford MGP took longer than one hour. Given the relatively small number of bookings carried out by each midwife compared to midwives in Ashford and Lewisham it is probable that the length of time spent by midwives was partly due to their lighter workload overall.

Duration of second and subsequent consultations across different locations

Table D.2 shows the time spent by the MGPs on second and subsequent consultations in different locations. The big difference between Ashford and Lewisham was that just over one third of the Ashford second and subsequent consultations were home-based (34 per cent) and two-thirds were GP practice-based (64 per cent), compared with Lewisham where over three-quarters of second and subsequent consultations were home-based (76 per cent) and less than one fifth had taken place at a GP practice (19 per cent).

Home-based consultations took, on average, 35.5 minutes in Lewisham compared to 38 minutes in Ashford, while consultations at GP practices took 23.8 minutes in Lewisham and 23.1 minutes in Ashford. 5 per cent of second and subsequent consultations in Lewisham took place in hospital compared with 2 per cent in Ashford.

The Deptford MGP was very different again in that the midwives did not carry out any second and subsequent consultations at GP practices. 69 per cent of the consultations were home-based, 19 per cent were carried out at the MGP office in the Community Centre, 2 per cent at midwives' own homes and the remainder in hospital. The Deptford MGP spent nearly twice as much time on home-based visits as the Lewisham MGP and 83 per cent more time than the Ashford MGP, while over twice as much time was spent on hospital visits by the Deptford MGP as in Lewisham or Ashford.

Table D.2 demonstrates the important resource implications involved in providing home-based consultations. Home-based second and subsequent consultations in Lewisham took 50 per cent more time than GP practice-based consultations and, in view of the total number of home-based consultations, this could be a matter of real concern.

Table D.2   Average length of time spent by MGPs on second and subsequent consultations in different locations

mean time in minutes

	Lewisham	Ashford	Deptford
Location			
Home	35.4	38.0	67.4
(Number of consultations)	(2350)	(929)	(613)
Hospital	58.7	58.2	92.5
(Number of consultations)	(144)	(45)	(66)
GP practice	23.8	23.1	15.0
(Number of consultations)	(597)	(1779)	(1)
Client's workplace	30.0	0	0
(Number of consultations)	(2)		
Midwife's home	0	0	75.6
(Number of consultations)		(17)	
Albany Centre	0	0	52.3
(Number of consultations)		(171)	
More than one location	57.5	43.8	179.2
(Number of consultations)	(2)	(4)	(19)
n.a.	(3)	(8)	(13)
All locations of second and subsequent consultations	*34.3*	*28.8*	*68.8*
(Number of consultations)	*(3098)*	*(2765)*	*(900)*

We calculated the time difference involved by looking at the total number and average length of home-based and GP practice-based consultations carried out during the monitoring period and found that this was 459 hours for the 18-month period. If midwives in Lewisham continue to spend 50 per cent longer on home-based consultations and carry out as many as three quarters of their consultations at home, the extra time commitment per annum required to maintain this would be equivalent to taking up one midwife's time (37.5 hours per week) for eight weeks.

In contrast, the Ashford MGP carried out two thirds of their second and subsequent consultations at GP practices which took 39 per cent less time than home-based consultations. The estimated time difference from this approach for the 18-month period was 411 hours. Similarly, if the MGP continues to carry out the same proportion of second and subsequent consultations in GP practices the amount of time saved by the MGP per annum would be equivalent to over seven weeks (37.5 hours per week) of one midwife's time.

We cannot comment on the different quality of home-based or GP practice-based consultations, but what is certain is that in looking at sustainable practice, the MGPs should become more aware of the implications of their particular approach to the organisation and provision of care. Any discussions should also take account of travel time and expenses incurred in providing home-based consultations.

Time spent by individual midwives on second and subsequent consultations in different locations

a) Home-based consultations: the average time spent by individual midwives on second and subsequent home-based consultations ranged from 26.1 minutes to 45.6 minutes in Lewisham, while in Ashford the time spent ranged from 25.3 to 56.4 minutes and in Deptford from 44.6 to 86 minutes.

b) Hospital-based consultations: second and subsequent consultations in hospital by the Lewisham MGP midwives ranged from 38.8 minutes to 82.5 minutes while in Ashford they ranged from 45 to 82.5 minutes and in Deptford from 38 to 172.1 minutes.

c) GP practice-based consultations: the average time spent on GP practice-based second and subsequent consultations in Lewisham ranged from 22.4 to 29.2 minutes and in Ashford from 18.1 to 29.1 minutes. GP practice-based consultations did not occur at all in Deptford.

There were also notable variations within the MGPs in relation to the proportion of consultations carried out in different locations by different midwives, with some midwives conducting a higher proportion of consultations in clients' homes than their colleagues. These findings raise a number of questions. Why do some midwives carry out more home-based consultations than others? What does this mean in terms of the care provided by different midwives to different women? Is it possible that the differences in location are entirely due to women's preferences or are variations also a result of the preferences of individual midwives and the way in which options are presented to women?

The length of hospital consultations is not surprising considering that many of these consultations were unscheduled and often associated with complications. The longer length of hospital consultations recorded by midwives in Deptford could be attributed to the fact that women were often accompanied by their midwife to specialist consultations and the time recorded invariably included a lengthy waiting time. Other hospital-based consultations were labour ward and delivery suite tours for women and their partners which would usually take longer than routine consultations.

It is noteworthy that the time spent by individual midwives on routine antenatal second and subsequent consultations could vary as markedly as we have seen between midwives from the same MGP. It is not surprising that midwives have different styles of working but, in view of the large differences observed, this may have a strong impact on the overall effectiveness of the MGPs.

The challenge for service providers in the future will be to strike a balance between presenting options for care, bearing in mind what can realistically be provided, so that there is not a mismatch between women's expressed wishes or preferences and the resources actually available. *Changing Childbirth* encourages professionals to tailor care to women's individual needs, but it also assumes that professionals will be aware of the wider implications of adopting certain approaches to the provision of care.

Appendix E

Interviews with women users of the midwifery group practices: sampling and methods

Personal interviews were carried out with 180 women who had booked with the midwifery group practices (MGPs) during the 18-month monitoring period from April 1994 to the end of September 1995. All interviews were carried out by members of the PSI research team or by two experienced interviewers. Semi-structured questionnaires were used for first and follow-up interviews. Respondents were asked the same questions in the same order, but a number of questions were 'open-ended' allowing for full answers to be recorded verbatim. Code-frames were constructed for the analysis of these answers. This technique allows for the extensive use of quotations from the interviews.

We aimed to carry out a total of 300 interviews with women – 180 first interviews and 120 follow-up interviews:

(i) 180 first interviews with women who had booked with the MGPs in April, July and October 1994, January, April and July 1995. Women who had booked with the Deptford MGP in intervening months were included when drawing up the sampling frames to ensure that each sampling period yielded a sufficient number of women to be interviewed. This was due to the small numbers who booked with this MGP and Table E.1 indicates that the low booking rate was particularly low during the October 1994 sampling period.

(ii) We planned to carry out follow-up interviews with 120 of the women who booked in the first 4 sampling periods. It was not initially planned that women who had booked in April or July 1995 would be included in follow-up interviews because it was assumed that they would not have delivered within the monitoring period. However, in the event we carried out follow-up interviews with 6 women who had booked with the MGPs in April and July 1995 because they had booked with the MGP at a late stage in pregnancy and had delivered before we could conduct a first interview with them.

Table E.1   Women interviewed during the 18-month monitoring period:
April 1994–September 1995

numbers

| | First interviews | | | | Second interviews | | | |
	Total	Lew	Ash	Dept	Total	Lew	Ash	Dept
Women booking in:								
April 1994	29	9	9	11	31	9	11	11
July 1994	36	12	12	12	34	12	11	11
October 1994	25	12	9	4	23	10	9	4
January 1995	30	11	9	10	23	8	9	6
April 1995	25	10	7	8	2	0	0	2
July 1995	23	8	9	6	4	1	1	2
Total: all women								
interviewed	*(168)**	*(62)*	*(55)*	*(51)*	*(117)*	*(40)*	*(41)*	*(36)*

*   In addition, 12 women had partial first interviews since they were interviewed after
delivery. They are included in the 117 second interviews.

PSI supplied letters to each MGP which were given to women by their
midwife at the first consultation or booking visit. The letter gave details of
the evaluation, stating that interviews with women would be carried out as
part of the study and that they might be chosen by random selection for
interview. At each sampling period PSI gave the MGP coordinator the
client numbers selected for interview. The names and addresses of women
were forwarded to PSI and women were contacted requesting an interview.
At the first interview, women who booked in April, July, October 1994
and January 1995 were asked if they would be willing to be interviewed
again around four weeks after delivery. The second interview was always
carried out by the same interviewer to ensure continuity.

i)   First interviews

Table E.1 shows the number of women who had first and follow-up interviews in all three areas. First interviews were carried out within three
months of booking with the MGPs. The refusal rate was 4 per cent. 62
first interviews were carried out with women who had booked with the
Lewisham MGP, 55 with women in Ashford and 51 with women in
Deptford.

ii)   Second follow-up interviews

119 women who had first interviews from sampling periods 1–4 were
asked if they would be willing to have a second follow-up interview, 105
of whom were subsequently interviewed after delivery. Of the 14 who did

not have follow-up interviews, 8 women had moved away during pregnancy or shortly after delivery, 3 women did not reply to the request for a second interview following delivery and in 3 cases the baby died or was unwell and the women did not have a follow-up interview.

In addition, 12 women had partial first interviews and full second interviews after delivery (3 women in Lewisham, 2 in Ashford and 6 women in Deptford). These women are included in the total of 117 in Table E.1 but not in the 168 first interviews in the table. This accounts for the smaller number of first interviews than second interviews in one of the sampling periods referred to in the table. Partial first interviews took place because women could not be contacted during pregnancy or had booked/transferred late to the MGPs. 40 women in Lewisham, 41 in Ashford and 36 in Deptford had follow-up or second interviews.

Overall, 180 women were interviewed: 168 full first interviews, 12 partial first interviews and 117 follow-up or second interviews.

Acronyms and abbreviations

ANC	Antenatal Clinic
DOMINO	Domiciliary In and Out
EDD	Expected Date of Delivery
EKHA	East Kent Health Authority
FCE	Finished Consultant Episode
FHSA	Family Health Services Authority
GP	General Practitioner
LSLHC	Lambeth, Southwark and Lewisham Health Commission
MGP	Midwifery Group Practice
NHS	National Health Service
PHCT	Primary Health Care Team
PSI	Policy Studies Institute
SETRHA	South East Thames Regional Health Authority
SHO	Senior House Officer
TENS	Transcutaneous Electronic Nerve Stimulation
TOP	Termination of Pregnancy

Recommended reading

Allen, I. (1991) *Family Planning and Pregnancy Counselling Projects for Young People.* London: Policy Studies Institute

Campbell, R. and Macfarlane, A. (1994) *Where To Be Born?* Oxford: National Perinatal Epidemiology Unit (second edition)

Chamberlain, G. and Patel, N. (eds) (1994) *The Future of the Maternity Services.* London: RCOG Press

Department of Health (1993) *Changing Childbirth.* Report of the Expert Maternity Group. London: HMSO

Dimond, B. (1994) *The Legal Aspects of Midwifery.* Cheshire: Books for Midwives Press

Enkin, M., Keirse, MJNC. and Chalmers, I. (1994) *A Guide to Effective Care in Pregnancy and Childbirth.* Oxford: Oxford University Press

Flint, C. (1993) *Midwifery Teams and Caseloads.* Oxford: Butterworth-Heinemann

Flint, C. and Poulengeris, P. (1987) *The Know Your Midwife Report.* 49 Peckerman's Wood, London SE6 6RZ

House of Commons Health Committee (1992) *Second Report, Maternity Services. Vols 1 and 2.* London: HMSO

Macfarlane, A., Mugford, M., Johnson, A. and Garcia, J. (1995) *Counting the Changes in Childbirth: Trends and Gaps in National Statistics.* Oxford: National Perinatal Epidemiology Unit

McCourt, C. and Page, L. (eds) (1996) *Report on the Evaluation of One-to-One Midwifery Practice.* London: Thames Valley University and Hammersmith Hospitals Trust

SETRHA (1994) *Maternity Services of the Future: The South East Thames Regional Health Authority Midwifery Group Practice Projects.* Nursing and Quality Directorate

SETRHA (1992) *Consensus Statement – Maternity Services of the Future.* Nursing and Quality Directorate

Wraight, A., Ball, J. and Seccombe, I. (1993) *Mapping Team Midwifery.* IMS Report Series 242. Brighton: Institute of Manpower Studies

Williams, S. and Allen I. (1989) *Health Care for Single Homeless People.* London: Policy Studies Institute